Carra / Hein

Englisch in der Apotheke

Englisch in der Apotheke

von Dagmar Carra und Martha Hein, München

5. Auflage

Deutscher Apotheker Verlag Stuttgart

Anschriften der Autorinnen

Dagmar Carra
Reischlweg 16
80939 München

Martha Hein
Rümannstraße 48
80804 München

Hinweise

Bibliografische Information der Deutschen Nationalbibliothek:
Die Deutsche Nationalbibliothek verzeichnet diese Publikation in der Deutschen Nationalbibliografie; detaillierte bibliografische Daten sind im Internet unter http://dnb.d-nb.de abrufbar.

ISBN 978-3-7692-4605-6

Birkenwaldstr. 44, 70191 Stuttgart
www.deutscher-apotheker-verlag.de
Printed in Germany
Satz: Werbung Gerd Kress, Stuttgart
Druck und Bindung: Kösel, Krugzell
Umschlagabbildung: khodjaev/fotolia
Umschlaggestaltung: deblik, Berlin

Vorwort

Das vorliegende Lehrwerk wendet sich an alle, die gelegentlich englischsprachige Kunden in der Apotheke bedienen, insbesondere an PTA. Somit ist sein Hauptaugenmerk auf die mündliche Kommunikation gerichtet.

Die Leser sollten über Grundkenntnisse in der englischen Sprache verfügen, wobei es von untergeordneter Bedeutung ist, wie umfangreich diese Sprachkenntnisse sind, denn durch die streng fachspezifische Orientierung werden die unterschiedlichen Voraussetzungen nivelliert.

Wir haben ein Buch konzipiert, das folgende Funktionen erfüllt:

- ☐ Durch die systematische Wortschatzarbeit in den ersten Kapiteln und die darauf abgestimmten Übungen dient es allen in der Apotheke Tätigen als fachspezifische Erweiterung vorhandener Englischkenntnisse. Anhand des knappen Grammatikteils, dessen Beispielsätze ebenfalls dem Apothekenalltag entnommen sind, können in Vergessenheit geratene Strukturen wieder aufgefrischt werden. Zu allen Übungen gibt es Lösungsvorschläge, die das Selbststudium erleichtern.
- ☐ Dank des ausführlichen Vokabelteils und der übersichtlich gegliederten „phrases“ in Kapitel 4 kann es als Nachschlagewerk in der Apotheke verwendet werden.
- ☐ Vor allem ist es aber als Lehrbuch für den Englischunterricht an PTA-Schulen gedacht. Sein Aufbau richtet sich nach dem in Bayern vorgeschriebenen Lehrplan. Die beiden Autorinnen haben ihre langjährige Unterrichtserfahrung an der Münchner PTA-Schule in das Buch mit eingebracht.

Unser besonderer Dank gilt Frau Rosemary FitzGibbon, die uns als native speaker bei der Überarbeitung der Texte des Lehrwerks sehr geholfen hat.

München, im Frühjahr 2008

Dagmar Carra und Martha Hein

Contents

The parts of the body | Die Teile des Körpers

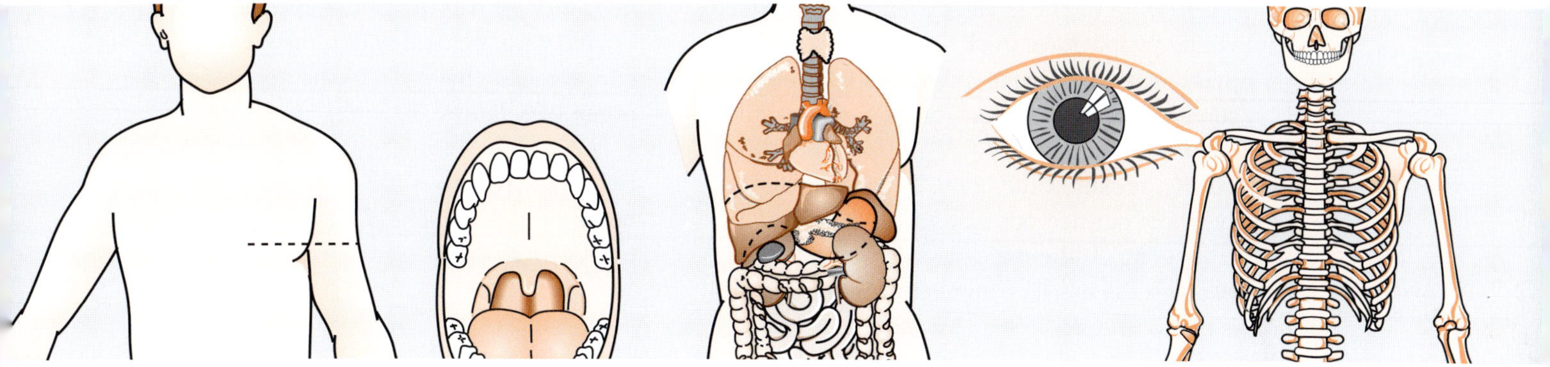

1

1.1. The head

The head consists of the face and the skull. The hair (*1) on the head can be fair or dark. Most young people have thick hair, either straight, perhaps with a parting, or curly. Older people sometimes have thin hair. Some men are bald.

Inside the skull is the brain, the coordinating centre of our nervous system. Each side of the brain controls the opposite side of the body. Beneath the hair-line and between the temples is the forehead.

We see with our (*2) eyes. The eyelids, the eyelashes and the eyebrows protect the eyes. People who cannot see well may be short-sighted or long-sighted. They have to wear glasses (*3). There are also people who are blind.

The nose with its two nostrils is the organ of smell. It is also important for the sense of taste. There are long noses, pointed or aquiline ones or snub noses.

The mouth forms the beginning of the alimentary canal. It is closed by the upper and the lower lip. Inside the mouth are the upper and the lower teeth with sixteen teeth (*4) in each jaw. The base of each tooth is covered by the gums. The tongue is an organ on the floor of the mouth with taste buds. It is important for taking in and swallowing food, and in articulating speech.

People hear with their ears. If someone cannot hear, if, e.g., his eardrum is seriously damaged, he is deaf. When he cannot speak, he is mute. People who are deaf and dumb can only communicate by signs. In the inner ear is the organ of balance.

Below the mouth is the chin. Some men grow a beard or a moustache. Others, however, prefer to be cleanshaven.

*1) The English usually use the word 'hair' in the singular (She has blond hair.), unless single hairs are meant (The old woman had three black hairs on her nose.).

*2) English-speaking people use the possessive pronoun more often than we do, in particular in connection with parts of the body. In German we say 'mit den Augen'.

*3) Glasses meaning the German word 'Brille' is always used in the plural.

*4) one tooth - 32 teeth

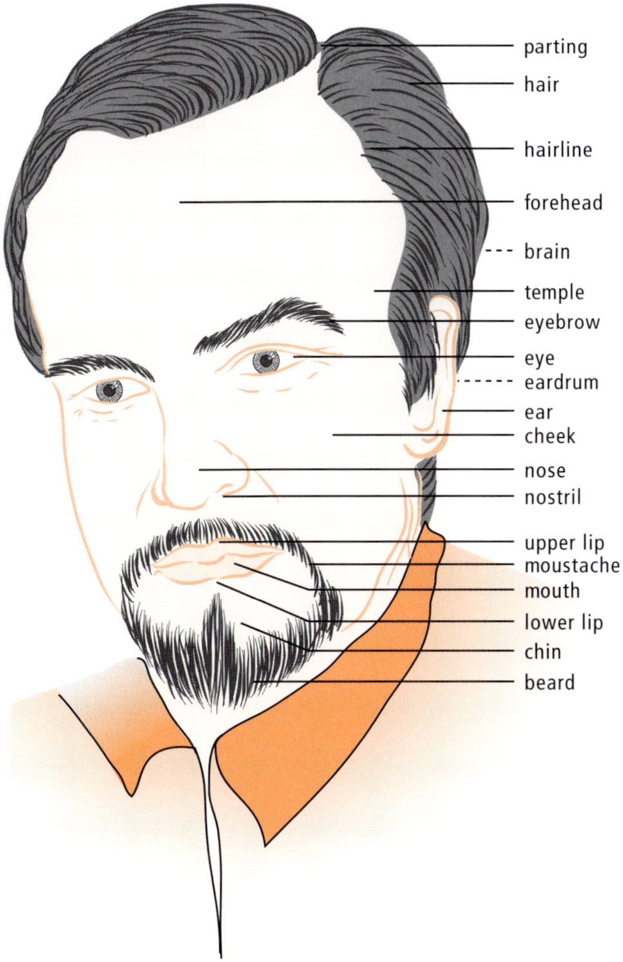

Fig. 1.1.: The head

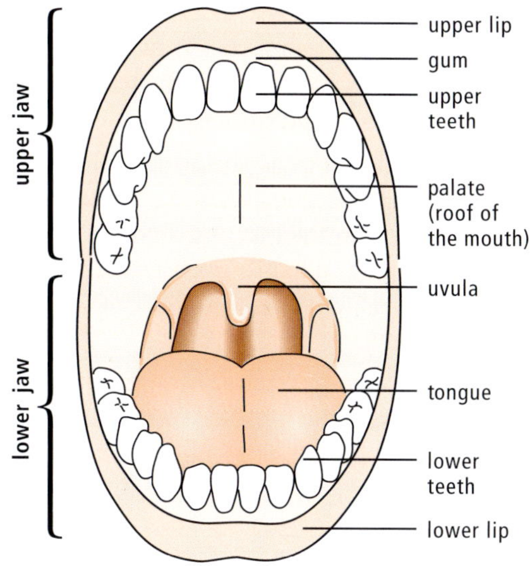

Fig. 1.2.: The mouth

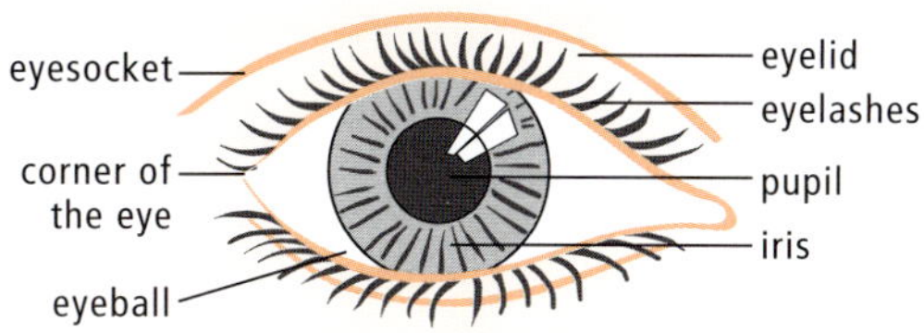

Fig. 1.3.: The eye

1.2. The trunk

*5) Little children often say 'tummy' instead of 'stomach'.

*6) Another word for 'abdomen' is 'belly'.

*7) The 'forefinger' can also be called 'index finger'.

*8) one calf - two calves

The neck connects the head and the trunk. Inside are the windpipe and the gullet, which lead to the lungs and the stomach(*5).

The trunk consists of the shoulders, the chest, the back, the buttocks and the abdomen (*6). Whereas a man's chest is flat, women have two breasts which secrete milk after childbirth.

The slimmest part of the trunk is the waist, which is above the hips. In the middle of the lower part of the abdomen is the navel.

1.3. The limbs

The limbs consist of the arms and the legs. An arm is made up of the upper arm, elbow, forearm, wrist and hand. On each hand we have a thumb and four fingers with fingernails: forefinger, middle finger, third finger and little finger (*7). The hand is remarkable for its flexibility. The thumb enables the hand to grasp objects.

The leg consists of the thigh, the knee, the shin (at the front) and the calf (at the back) (*8), the ankle, which can be sprained so easily, and the foot (*9). Each foot has a heel, a sole and five toes. A lot of people suffer from flat feet and therefore have to wear supports.

*9) one foot - two feet
The length of a man's foot was originally taken as a unit of linear measure:

1 inch (in)	=		2,54 cm
1 foot (ft)	=	12 in	= 30,48 cm
1 yard (yd)	=	3 ft	= 91,44 cm

Fig. 1.4.: The trunk and the limbs

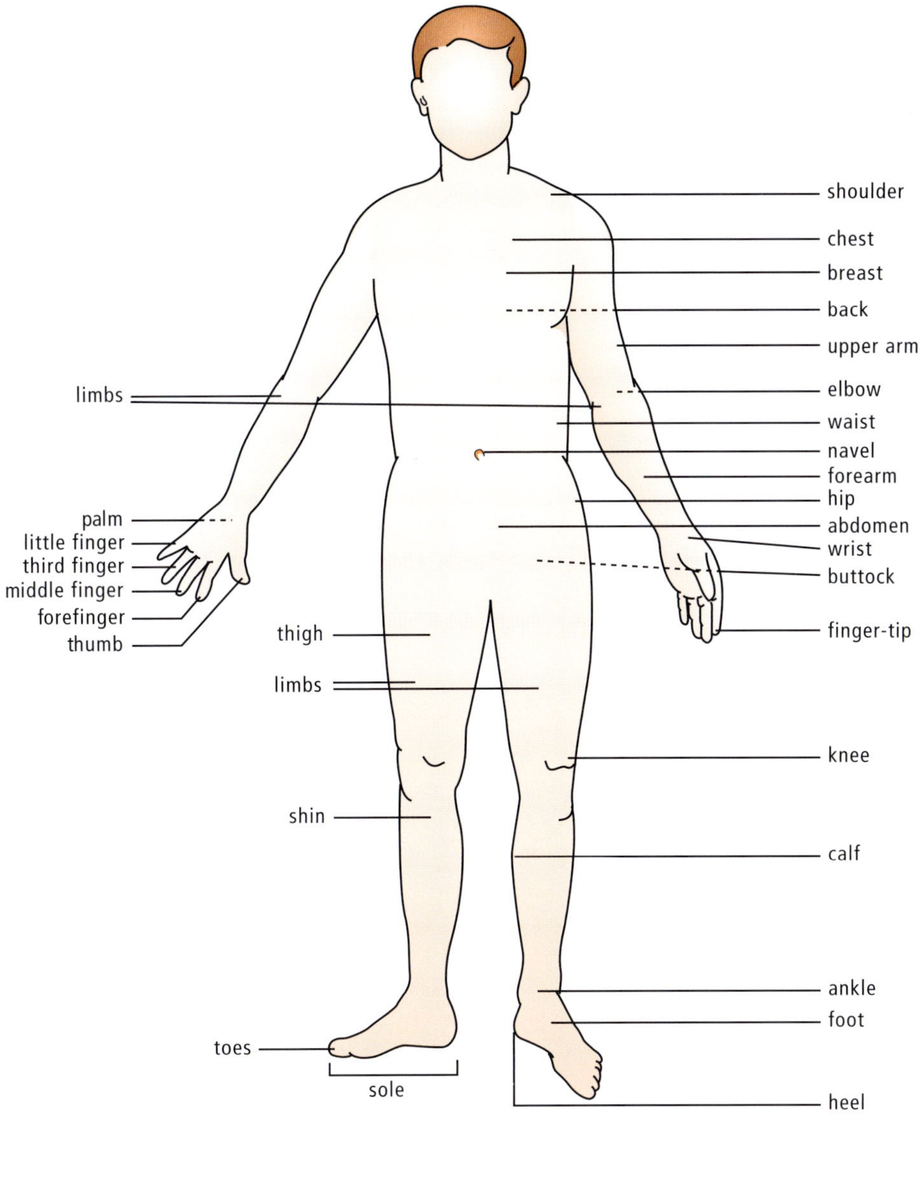

1.4. The skin

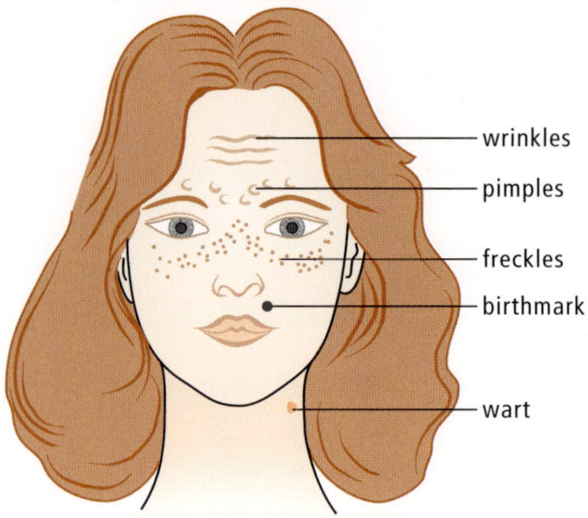

Fig. 1.5.: The skin

The skin is the tissue which forms the outer covering of the body. Whereas a baby's skin is smooth, boys and girls during puberty often have pimples. Older people often get wrinkles. A birthmark is a mark we have had since birth. Warts, however, are small, hard outgrowths on the skin which usually develop through a viral infection. Red-haired people, in particular, often get freckles on their noses and cheeks in the sun. When we are in good health our complexion is rosy. When we are ill, we look pale.

1.5. The skeleton

The skeleton gives structure to the body and protects the internal organs. The spine or backbone (*10) is the central part of the human skeleton. Among the other important bones are the shoulder-blades, the ribs, the breastbone, the radius and the ulna, the hipbone, the knee-cap and the shin-bone.

*10) Another word for 'spine' or 'backbone' is 'vertebral column'. A vertebra is one of its bony joints or segments.

All long bones contain bone-marrow. The place where bones are connected are called joints. The sinews or tendons attach the muscles to the bones. They should not be confused with ligaments, which hold bones together to keep them in the right place.

Fig. 1.6.: The skeleton

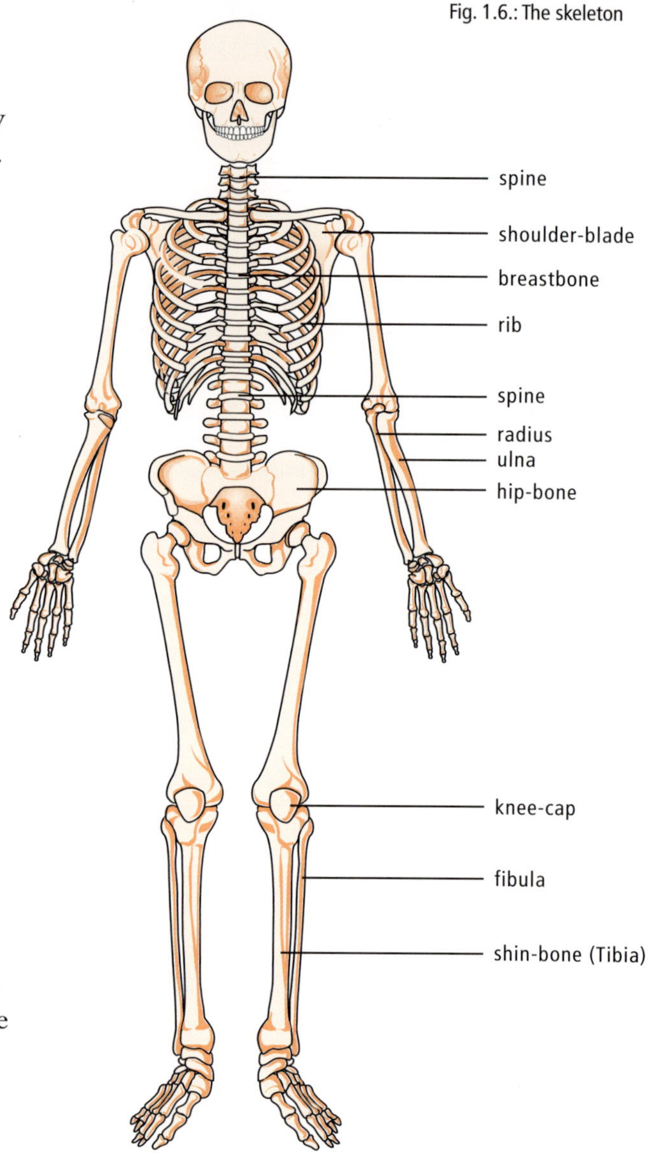

1.6. Some internal organs

Inside the chest are the heart and lungs, protected by the ribs. The heart is the pump that keeps the blood moving in the blood vessels. Blood is carried from the heart to all parts of the body by way of arteries. It travels back to the heart in the veins. It is purified by the liver and the kidneys. The liver is the largest gland of the body. It secretes bile, which is stored in the gall bladder. Bile allows the body to digest fat and helps it to absorb vitamins A, D, E and K. The liver has additional tasks, such as the regulation of the sugar content of the blood under the influence of insulin, a hormone secreted by the pancreas. The kidneys are bean-shaped organs that also regulate salt and fluid levels in the body. Another organ that helps to make the blood pure is the spleen, which is situated to the left of the stomach. The digestive tract is over 30 ft long, beginning in the mouth and ending in the anus. It includes the gullet, the stomach and the intestines, which are divided into the small intestine and the large intestine (*11).

*11) Another word for the 'intestines' is 'gut'.

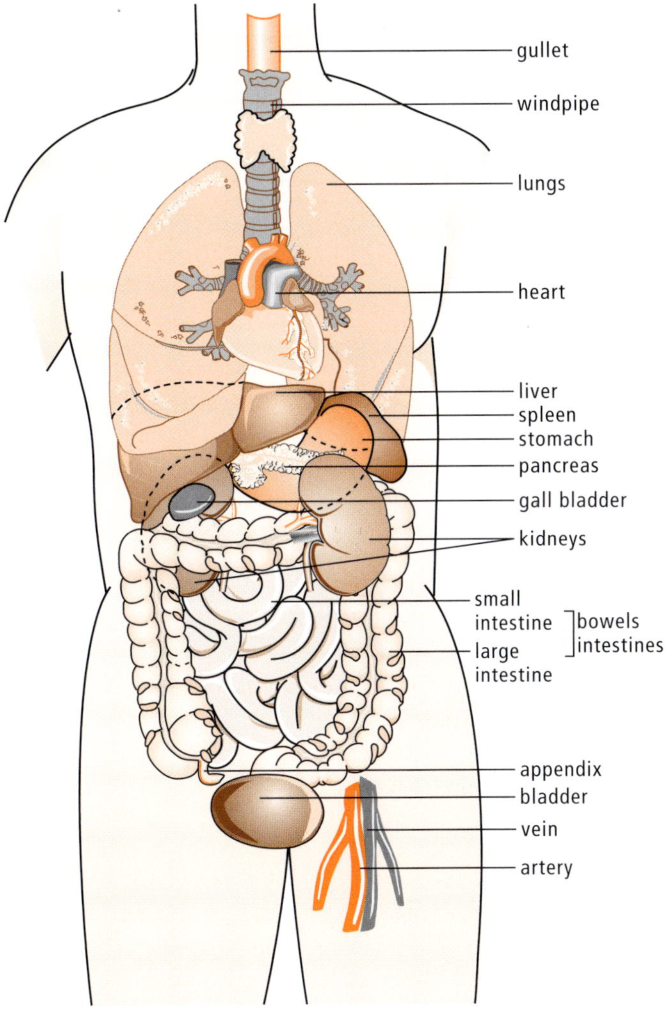

Fig. 1.7.: The internal organs

✳ Übungen zu Kapitel 1 ab Seite 48.

Illnesses and injuries | Krankheiten und Verletzungen

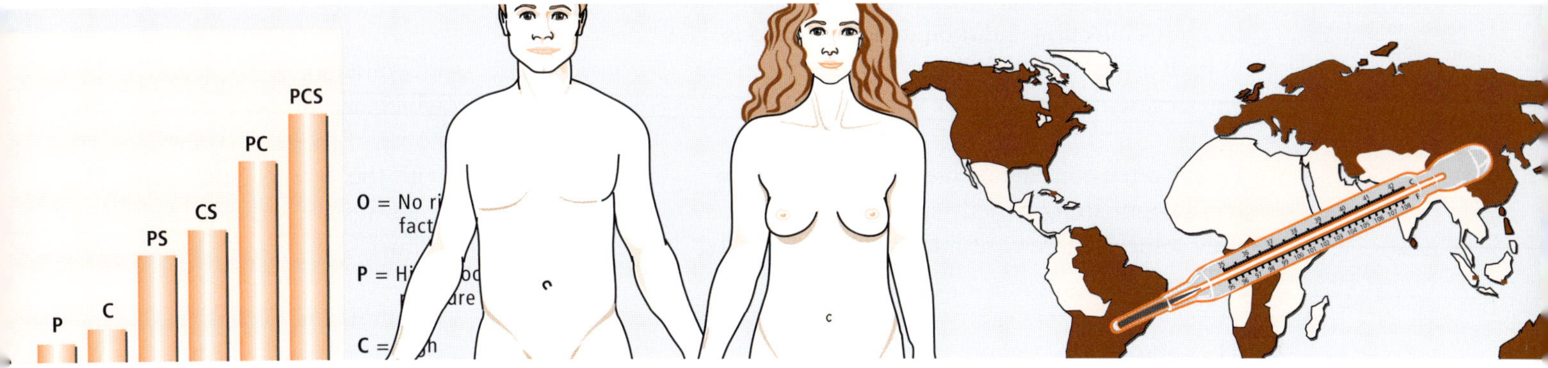

2

2.1. Coughs and colds

The common cold is a general term for one of the most frequent minor illnesses (*1). It is due to a virus infection and though not dangerous in itself it is often the forerunner of more serious illnesses, some of which are described below.

People often consider a cold and the flu (*2) to be the same thing. Strictly speaking, however, only some of these virus infections can be called influenza.

They sometimes become epidemics like "Spanish flu", which affected over 500 million people between 1918 and 1922, 22 million of whom died.

General signs of colds are:
headache (*3), hoarseness, weariness, catarrh, cough, and, in the case of fever, shivering fits.

More serious side effects of the common cold, amongst others, are:

sinusitis (*4):	inflammation of the sinuses, which are hollow cavities in the bones of the skull connecting with the nasal cavities. Sinusitis is always accompanied by catarrh.
tonsillitis:	inflammation of the tonsils, which become swollen as a result of bacterial or viral infection.
bronchitis:	inflammation of the bronchial tubes (*5). Usually a cough mixture or syrup will bring relief. Severe cases, however, might lead to pneumonia.
pneumonia:	inflammation of the lung. There are various types of pneumonia, all of which can be very serious and require careful nursing in bed.

*1) Synonyms for 'illness' are 'sickness' and 'ailment'.

*2) 'Flu' is a frequently used abbreviation for 'influenza'.

*3) 'Ache' is a synonym for 'pain' and occurs in words like 'toothache', 'backache', 'stomachache' etc.

*4) The ending '-itis' means 'inflammation'. Other examples: appendicitis, tonsillitis, bronchitis, poliomyelitis, nephritis.

*5) A synonym is 'bronchi'.

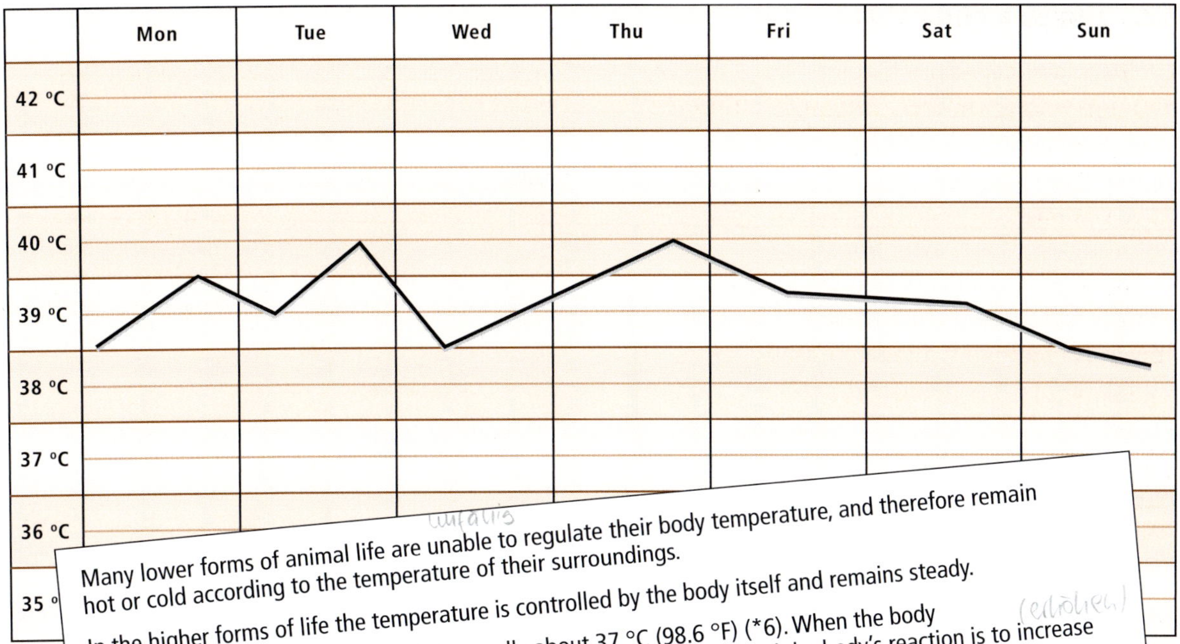

Many lower forms of animal life are unable to regulate their body temperature, and therefore remain hot or cold according to the temperature of their surroundings.

In the higher forms of life the temperature is controlled by the body itself and remains steady.

The temperature of the human body is usually about 37 °C (98.6 °F) (*6). When the body is attacked by germs a complicated defence system comes into play, and the body's reaction is to increase the temperature. A child's temperature may vary during the day. It can be raised by excitement, incessant crying or running about.

But any temperature over 38 °C (100.4 °F) is classed as a fever.

Fig. 2.1.: Thermometer

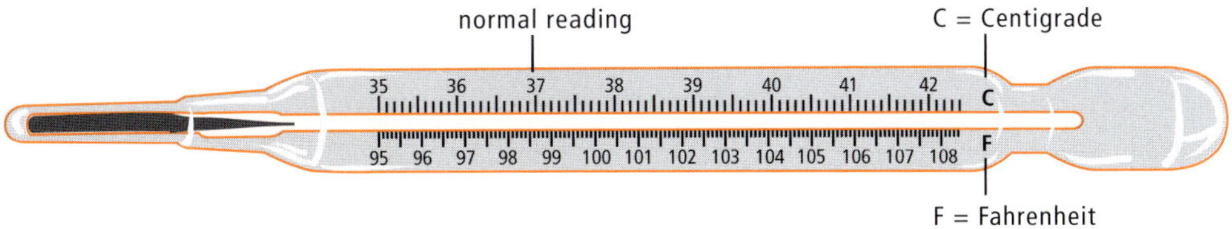

*6) In English-speaking countries the unit of temperature is 1 degree Fahrenheit. The Fahrenheit thermometric scale extends from 0° to 212°.
0° F = –18°C;
32° F = 0°C (freezing point);
212° F = 100° C (boiling point)

To convert from Fahrenheit into Centigrade we substract 32, multiply by 5 and divide by 9.
To convert from Centigrade into Fahrenheit we mulitply by 9, divide by 5 and add 32.
Example: 30°C:
30 × 9 = 270
270 : 5 = 54
54+32 = 86
30°C = 86° F

The English put a decimal point when writing 98.8; on the other hand they put commas in 1,000,000.

2.2. The sick child (*7)

There are a few illnesses that are common among children. Although most of them are not dangerous, they should not be ignored.

Disturbing signs and symptoms accompany some of these ailments. In many infections a child sweats, shivers, runs a high temperature, and is tired, flushed, apathetic and has no appetite. A rash or spots appear in scarlet fever, measles and German measles. Diarrhoea and vomiting may result from a variety of causes. Sore throats accompany diphtheria, mononucleosis and poliomyelitis. Aching and shivering accompany mumps, chickenpox and German measles. But many of these signs and symptoms are not serious and vanish overnight.

7) sick and ill:
The sick boy...
Der kranke Junge...
The boy is ill...
Der Junge ist krank...
The boy is being sick.
The boy is vomiting
(= Der Junge muss sich übergeben).
In American English 'sick' is often used to mean 'ill'.

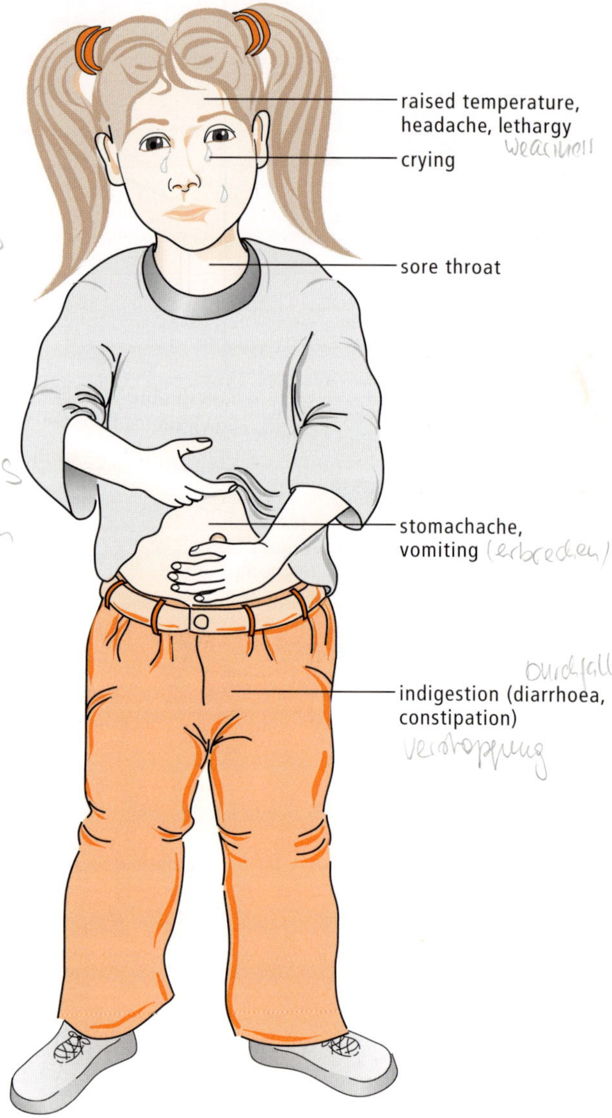

Some of the most frequent children's illnesses are accompanied by a rash:

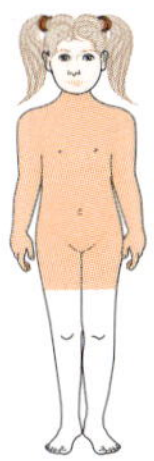

In measles a rash develops on the third to the fifth day of the illness. Often it begins behind the ears and then spreads over the body

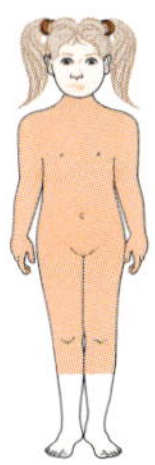

German measles is accompanied by a light pink rash. The spots often merge to give a flushed appearance.

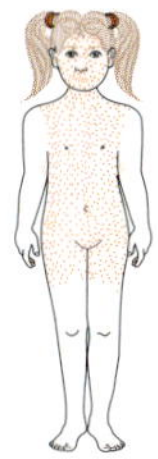

In chickenpox a rash is often the first sign of illness. It consists of dark red pimples on which blisters develop after a few hours.

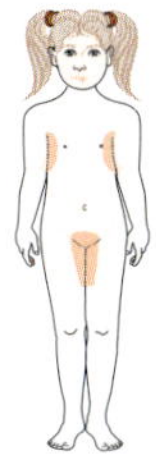

In scarlet fever a rash spreads over the body from damp areas like the armpits, the groin etc.

2.3. Vaccination

Vaccination can protect children against many diseases which once caused death and disabilities. In Germany paediatricians (*8) recommend the following vaccination programme for children:

Fig. 2.4.: Vaccination programme

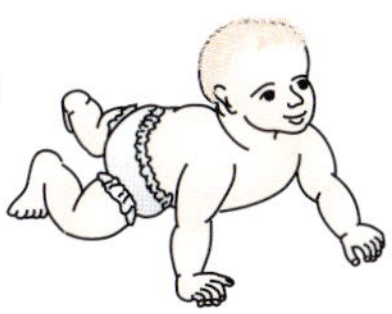

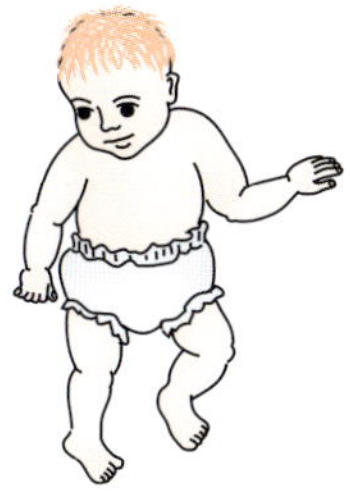

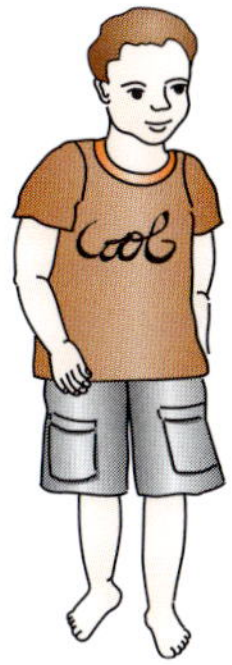

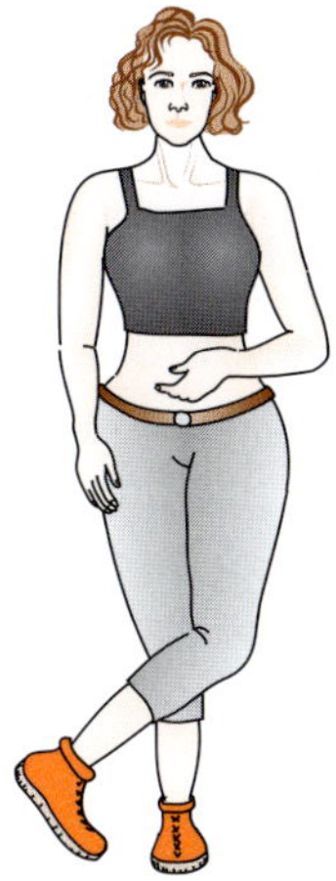

2–4 Months	11–14 Months		5–6 Years	9–17 Years
polio diphtheria tetanus whooping cough haemophilus influenzae b hepatitis B	polio diphtheria tetanus whooping cough haemophilus influenzae b hepatitis B measles	mumps German measles varicella (chickenpox)	diphtheria (booster) tetanus (booster)	polio (booster) tetanus (booster) diphtheria (booster) whooping cough (booster)

*8) Other specialists

neurologist	Neurologe	surgeon	Chirurg	psychiatrist	Psychiater
oculist	Augenarzt	dermatologist	Hautarzt	general practitioner	Allgemeinmediziner
orthopaedist	Orthopäde	gynaecologist	Frauenarzt		

2.4. Cardiovascular disorders

Diseases of the heart occur more often in rich societies than in developing countries.

A serious heart attack or coronary thrombosis can cause cardiac infarction or death of tissue because the blood supply has been cut off.

Risk factors associated with heart trouble include high cholesterol level, high blood pressure, being overweight and cigarette smoking. Another important factor that increases the risk of a heart attack is, of course, age. Dangerous as heart attacks are they do not necessarily cause death (*9).

*9) A serious medical condition in which the heart does not work correctly can also be called heart failure.

If the blood supply to the brain is reduced e. g. by thromboses (*10) or embolisms, this might lead to a stroke (*11).

*10) A thrombosis – several thromboses
*11) A medical term for stroke is apoplectic fit.

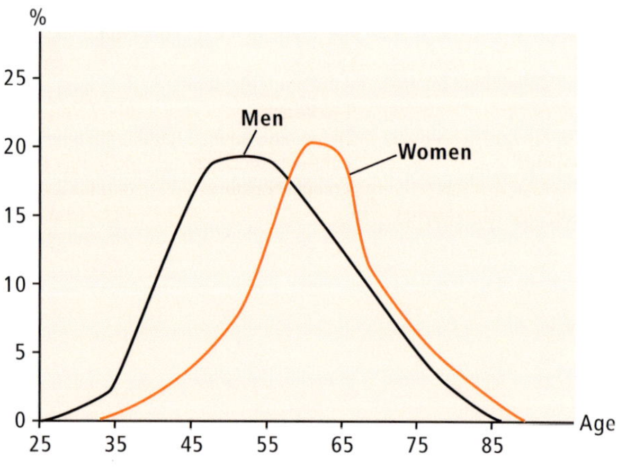

Fig. 2.6.: Frequency of cardiac infarctions in men and women

Strokes are more common in men than in women. They can vary in severity causing unconsciousness, paralysis and possibly death.

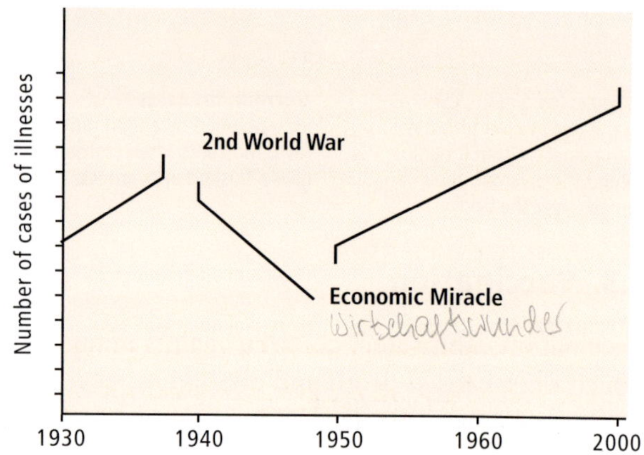

Fig. 2.5.: Frequency of cardiac infarctions in Germany during the last seventy years

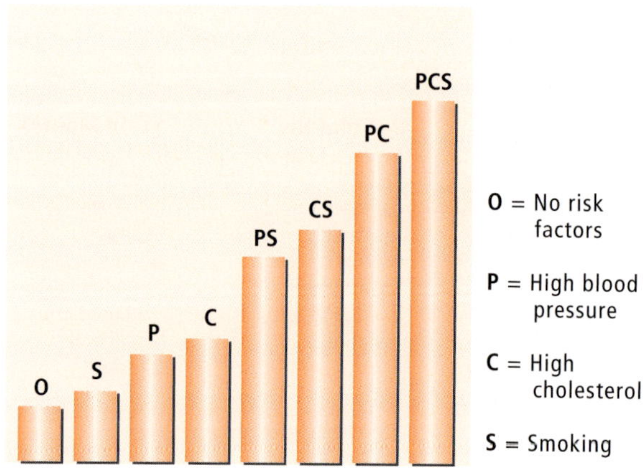

Fig. 2.7.: Relative risk of a cardiac infarction in a 50-year-old man

Other heart and circulatory disorders are
- □ constriction of the heart, that occurs in angina pectoris,
- □ circulatory or heart failure, caused by too little output of blood,
- □ congenital heart disease, which often requires an operation,
- □ varicose veins, which are more common in older people and in women who are pregnant,
- □ irregularities of the heartbeat (*12).

*12) A minor problem connected with blood circulation is nosebleed, i.e. bleeding from the nose, usually caused by a blow or by sneezing or by high blood pressure. Heartburn, however, is no circulatory problem but is caused by indigestion.

Fig. 2.8.: Thrombosis and embolism

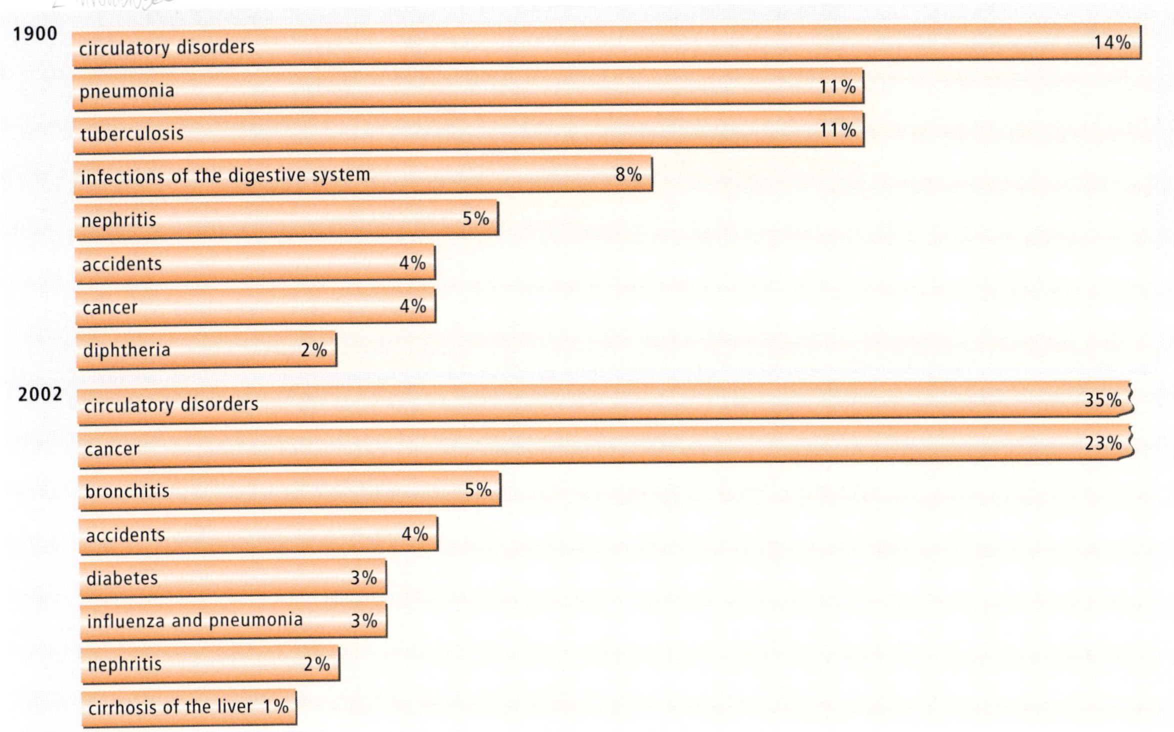

Fig. 2.9.: Causes of death in the USA in 1900 and 2002

2.5. Cancers

Whereas at the beginning of the twentieth century only 64 out of 100,000 inhabitants in Germany suffered from cancer it has now become the second most common disease. One reason might be that life expectancy used to be much lower and people died of other diseases.

Cancer is a tumour (*13) or growth of body tissue that may become malignant (*14). It can grow almost anywhere in the body, the most frequent sites being listed in fig. 2.10.

*14) The opposite of 'malignant' is 'benign'.

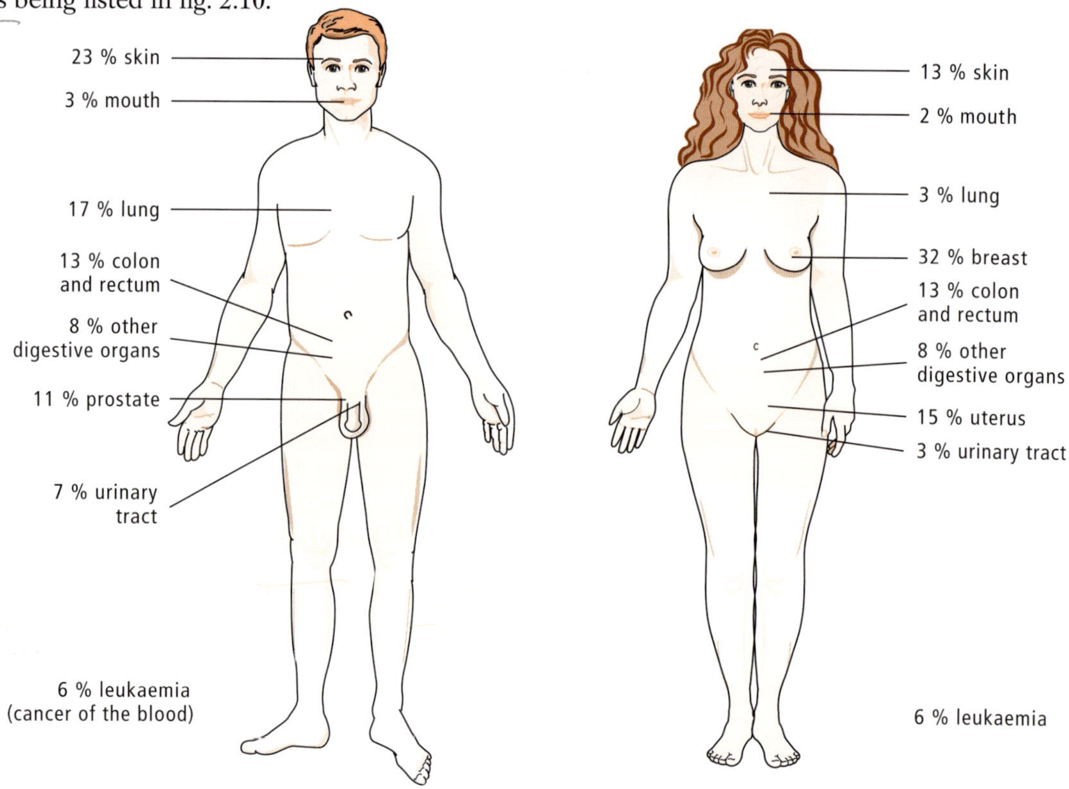

Fig. 2.10.: Common cancer sites in the body

2.6. Tropical diseases

Tropical diseases are on the increase in Central Europe. This is due to the increasing amount of travel to the tropics and the carelessness of many tourists, who do not bother to take any precautions against tropical diseases.

*13) Americans spell some words differently, e.g.

tumor	instead of	tumour,
diarrhea	instead of	diarrhoea,
leukemia	instead of	leukaemia,
orthopedist	instead of	orthopaedist etc.

The following leaflet used to be handed out at Munich Airport:

BAYERISCHES STAATSMINISTERIUM DES INNEREN

Cholera

You have entered Germany from a country in which some cases of cholera have occurred. We therefore ask you to take the following precautions in your own interest:

Cholera is an infectious disease of the intestine. The incubation period, i. e. the time between exposure to infection and the appearance of the first symptoms, is five days. Should you be affected by diarrhoea after your arrival, you must immediately consult a doctor and mention your recent stay abroad. You should then avoid any contact with other persons. We would also recommend careful personal hygiene.

Infectious diseases like cholera cause death in poorer parts of the world. Fig. 2.11. shows the spread of diseases like typhoid (*15), cholera, dysentery, tuberculosis, meningitis, smallpox, yellow fever, malaria etc.

Cardiovascular disorders and cancers, on the other hand, are more of a problem in affluent countries, as the maps in fig. 2.12. and fig. 2.13. show.

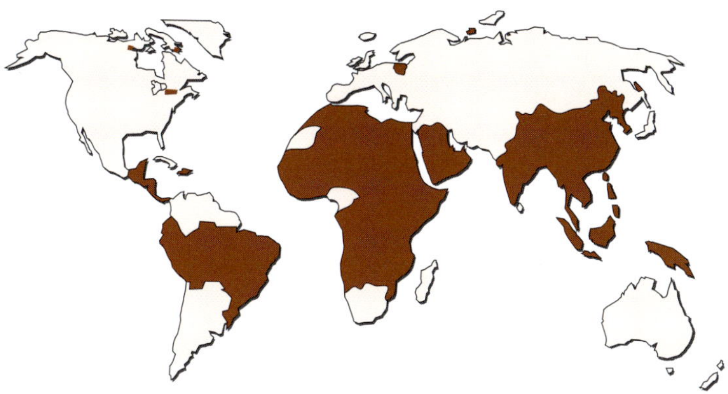

Fig. 2.11.: Causes of death: Infectious diseases

*15) “Typhoid” or “typhoid fever” means “Typhus” in German, whereas the meaning of the English word “typhus” is “Fleckfieber”.

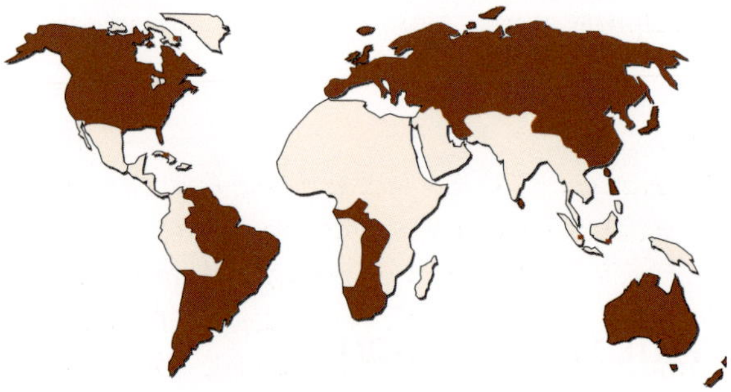

Fig. 2.12.: Causes of death: Cardiovascular disorders

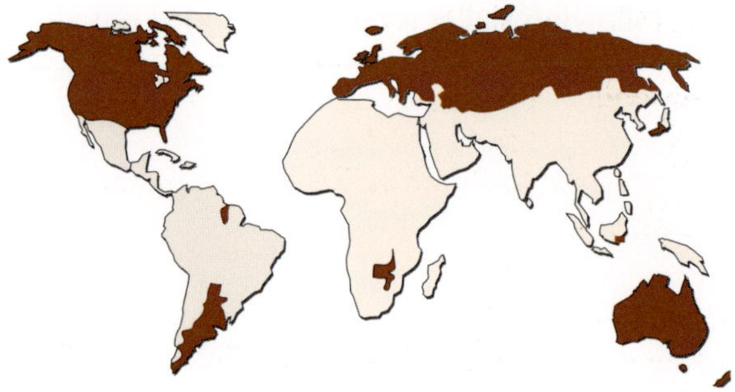

Fig. 2.13.: Causes of death: Cancer

2.7. Additional illnesses

The following "Medical advice page" in HEALTH-Magazine will make you familiar with other illnesses of various kinds:

MEDICAL ADVICE PAGE

Topic of the week: HOLIDAYS

In a couple of weeks the summer holidays will start and thousands of people will travel South. Are you prepared?
Don't forget to take a remedy for travel-sickness or sea-sickness, if you are prone to suffer from these problems.
Remember that the sun can cause significant damage, if you don't obey certain rules. Don't stay in the sun too long, particularly during the first few days. A reddening or blistering of the skin is a sign of sunburn. Sunstroke can be a more serious result of over-exposure to the sun without adequate cover for the head. The first symptom is often a bad headache.
If the headache is accompanied by cardiac insufficiency, leading to unconsciousness, this points to heatstroke and a doctor must be called immediately.

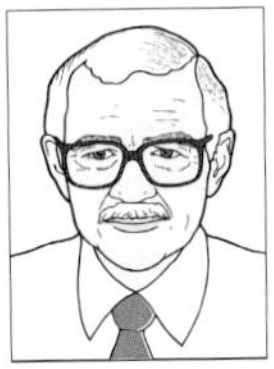

Ask Dr Scott
If you have a problem, don't hesitate to consult Dr Scott, HEALTH-Magazine, 40 Primrose Rd., Birmingham

*Dear Dr Scott (*16),*
*Every (*17) year in early summer I feel terrible. I suffer from sleeplessness, goose-pimples and, what's worse, difficulty in breathing. My brother told me that adenoids make breathing difficult. Is that true?*
Yours sincerely, John Baker

Dear Mr Baker,
Adenoids are a collection of lymphoid tissue at the back of the nose. They can obstruct breathing through the nose, in particular in children. As your problems occur every year at the same time, I suspect you suffer from an allergy to certain pollens. Please ask your doctor to examine you for allergic reactions. Sleeplessness and goose-pimples might stem from the fear of not being able to breathe properly.

Dear Dr Scott,
Our 15-year-old daughter occasionally suffers from severe abdominal pains. We tried to find out whether they were due to certain kinds of food which don't agree with her – without any success.
Sincerely yours, Jane Morton

Dear Mrs Morton,
It is very difficult to give you an adequate explanation. Your description is too vague. Are you sure your daughter does not suffer from period pains, which can be quite agonizing at her age? If not, she should really consult a doctor to rule out a more serious problem such as gall stones.

Dear Dr Scott,
My husband (53) has been suffering from painful rheumatism for over 9 months now. He is a lorrydriver and often has to carry heavy weights. During the last few weeks he has suffered from attacks of lumbago whenever he had to lift a heavy parcel. About 5 years ago he had problems with sciatica.
Sincerely yours, Carol Miller

Dear Mrs Miller,
Backache has become one of the most common complaints. There are some simple rules for looking after one's back, such as standing close to the object one wants to lift, with one's feet apart, the knees bent and the back straight. I am sure your doctor can give you a leaflet with useful advice. I would suggest your husband learns to do some special exercises for the back and, just as important, how to relax.

Dear Dr Scott,
I'm four months pregnant and suffer from painful piles. My sister told me that they will have to be removed in hospital. Is that true?
Yours sincerely, Brenda Simpson

Dear Mrs Simpson,
Don't worry. Haemorrhoids or piles often occur during pregnancy, and usually disappear after a few weeks. Your doctor can prescribe some ointment which will bring you relief.

*16) In German we say 'Herr Dr. X', in English just 'Dr X.'

*17) The first word in a letter always starts with a capital letter.

2.8. Injuries

Have a look at the following story about poor Stephen's unlucky day and learn some important terms to do with injuries:

Five minutes to nine. Stephen was extremely late for work this morning. He had run all the way from home to Birchtree Road, so that he had a painful stitch in his side. Bathed in sweat he crossed the street. Suddenly, a blue Ford was in front of him. Neither of them could stop. When Stephen regained consciousness he found himself in the X-ray department at St. Mary's Hospital. "Is my leg broken?" he asked the nurse who stood beside his bed.

"Yes, my dear", she answered, "but I'm afraid that's not all, a muscle in your right forearm is torn, another one strained. I guess you'll have to be operated on to prevent stiffness. And look at all the bruises and skin abrasions, poor thing." "This terrible headache," Stephen moaned. "You might be suffering from concussion," the nurse explained. "But don't worry, in a couple of weeks you will have forgotten all about your injuries. In the meantime we'll do all we can for you".

When Stephen's wife arrived at the hospital she had to fill in the following form for him:

ST. MARY'S HOSPITAL + ADMISSION CARD

surname: ______
first name: ______
address and telephone number: ______
______
______
date of birth: ______
marital status: ______
married/single/widowed/divorced/other
occupation: ______
______
name and address of next of kin: ______
______
______
______
______
name and address of G.P.: ______
______
______
______

Have you ever had (please tick yes or no)

German measles	yes	no
venereal diseases	yes	no
date: ______		
high blood pressure	yes	no
varicose veins	yes	no
migraine	yes	no
heart trouble	yes	no
kidney or bladder problems	yes	no
diabetes	yes	no
epilepsy	yes	no
hepatitis	yes	no
date: ______		
cancer	yes	no
psychiatric treatment	yes	no
any serious illness: ______		

______
______

Have you ever had an operation?	yes	no
If yes, what type of operation and when? ______		
Do you take any medicine regularly?	yes	no
If so, what? ______		
Allergies to medications?	yes	no
If so, what? ______		
Do you smoke?	yes	no
How many per day? ______		
Do you have any mental problems in your family?	yes	no
If yes, what type of problems? ______		
What health problems run in your family? ______		

After a few days Stephen was allowed to get up and move around in a wheelchair. He met lots of other patients:

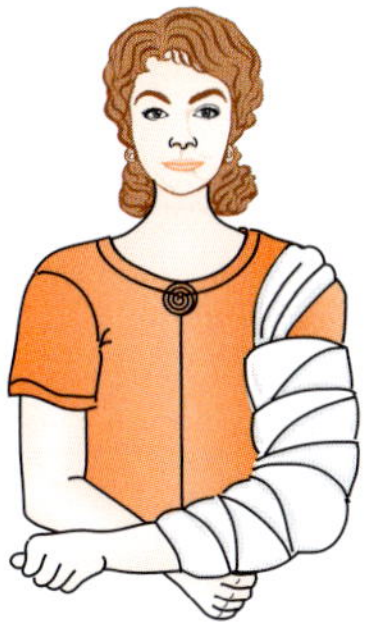

Sally fell asleep while smoking a cigarette in bed. She has severe burns all over her left arm.

Ben plays football every Saturday. He suffered a rupture of a muscle fibre in his last match.

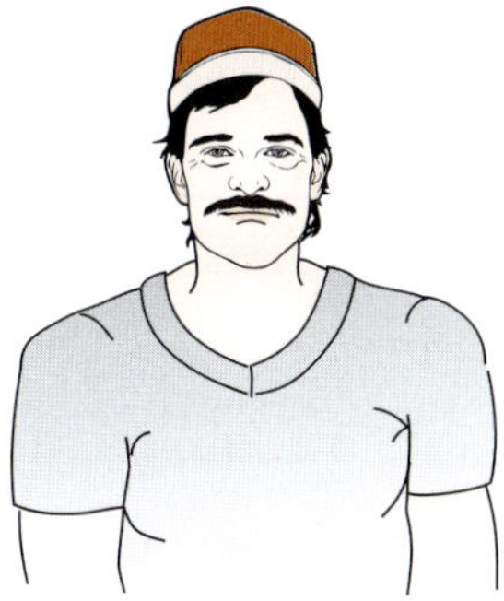

Richard, an enthusiastic tennis player, was tormented by cramps in his leg. In spite of this he went on playing. He made an unfortunate movement and tore a ligament.

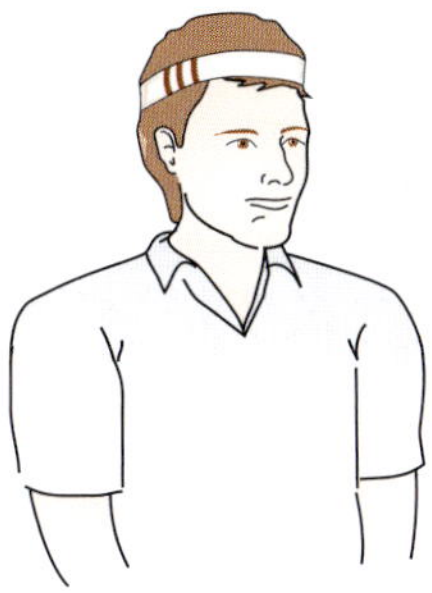

Charles fell off a ladder. He sprained his ankle and dislocated his left shoulder.

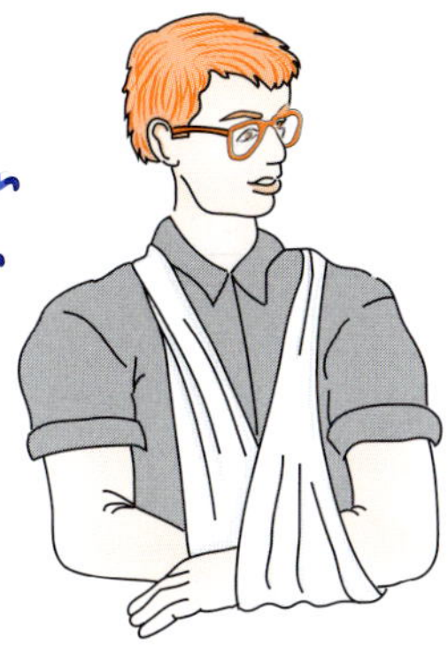

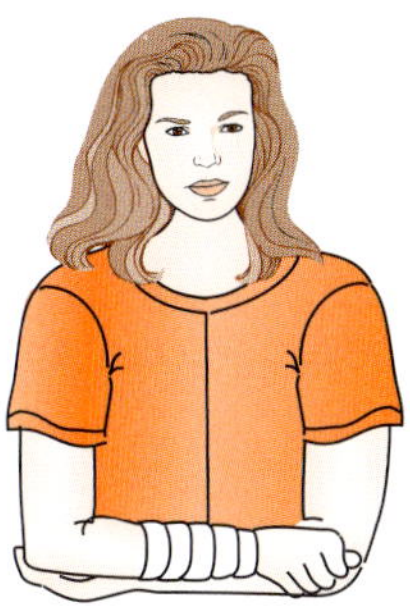

Mary is a secretary and has been troubled by inflammation of a tendon. She is an outpatient at St. Mary's.

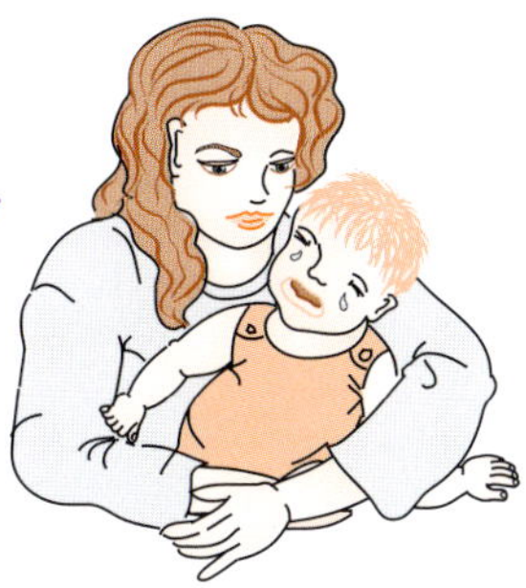

Billy was stung or bitten by an insect and is crying. He is waiting with his mother in the outpatients department.

✳ Übungen zu Kapitel 2 ab Seite 50.

Remedies and other articles sold at the chemist's

Arzneimittel und apothekenübliche Waren

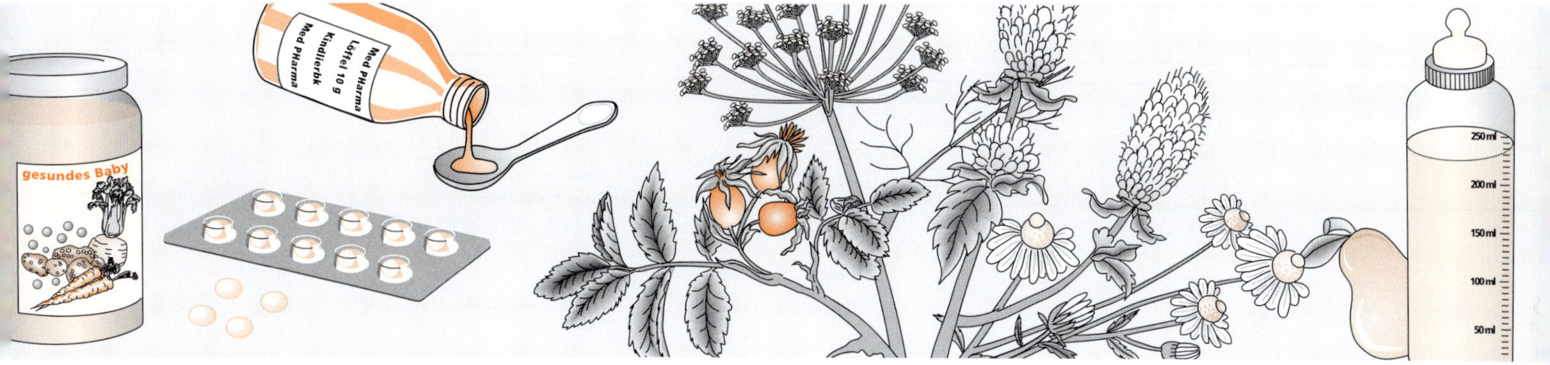

3

3.1. Some common remedies

Every year in spring Mrs Miller catches a cold. Her friends have lots of advice for her:

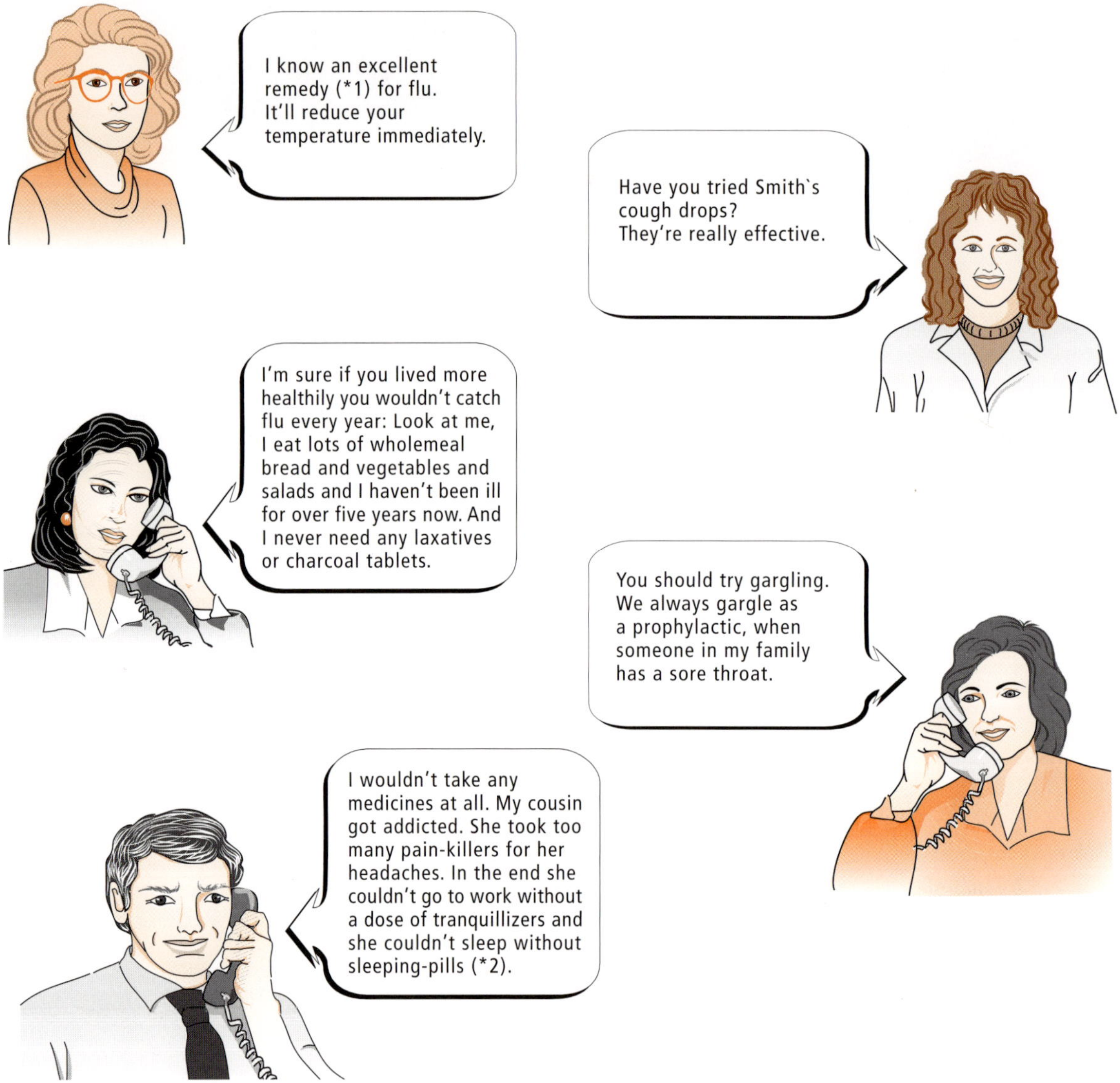
I know an excellent remedy (*1) for flu. It'll reduce your temperature immediately.
Have you tried Smith`s cough drops? They're really effective.
I'm sure if you lived more healthily you wouldn't catch flu every year: Look at me, I eat lots of wholemeal bread and vegetables and salads and I haven't been ill for over five years now. And I never need any laxatives or charcoal tablets.
You should try gargling. We always gargle as a prophylactic, when someone in my family has a sore throat.
I wouldn't take any medicines at all. My cousin got addicted. She took too many pain-killers for her headaches. In the end she couldn't go to work without a dose of tranquillizers and she couldn't sleep without sleeping-pills (*2).

*1) Another expression for 'remedy' is 'medicine'. In German we say 'Ein Medikament gegen...', whereas in English we say 'A remedy for...' Some remedies are only available on prescription, while others are sold over the counter.

*2) Another word for 'tranquillizer' is 'sedative', and instead of 'sleeping-pills' you can say 'tablets for insomnia'.

Customers usually have a very limited knowledge of pharmacology. They just know that there are

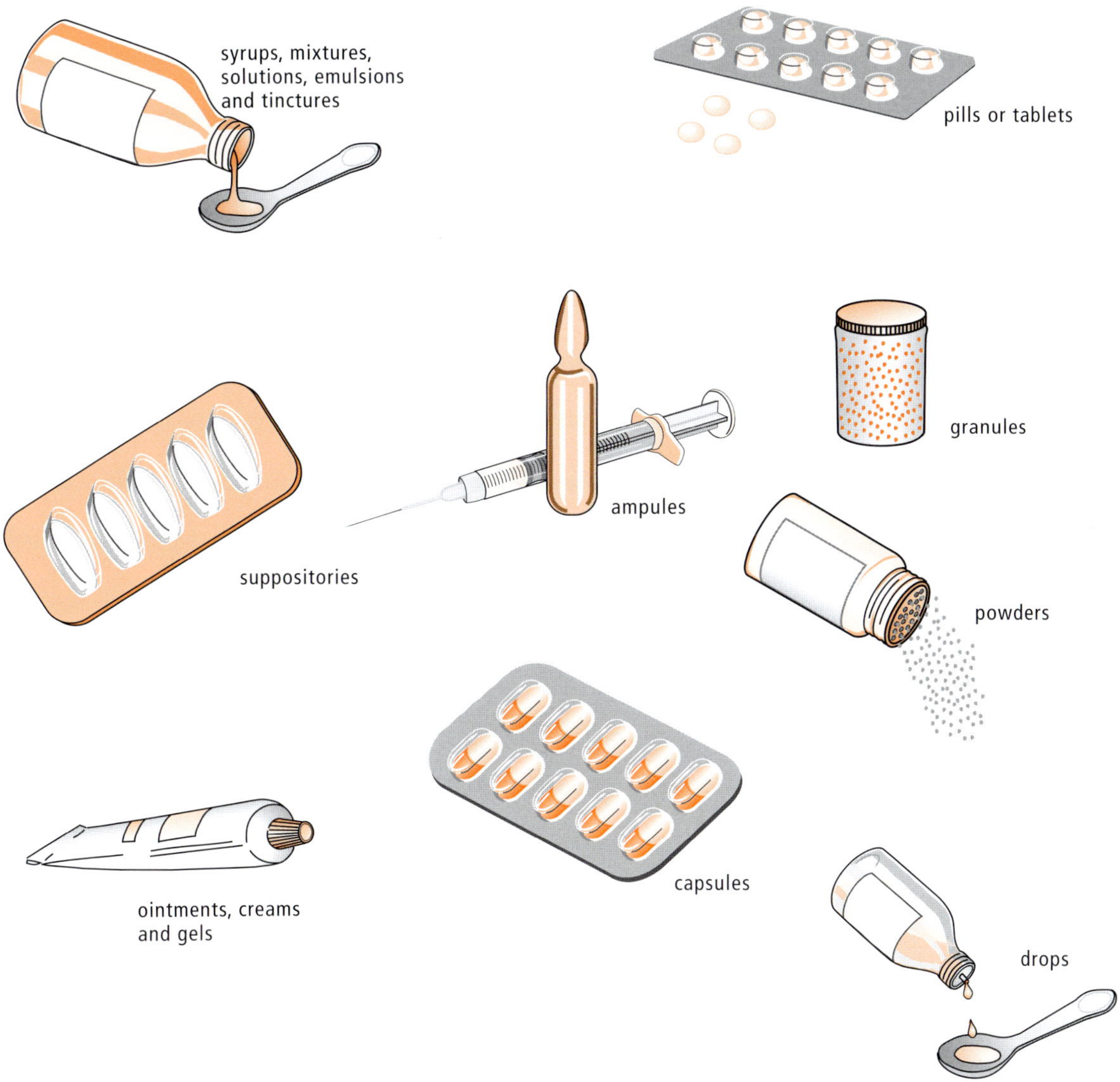

Fig. 3.1.: Various kinds of remedies

3.2. Methods of administration

The following table shows a more detailed list of different methods of administration:

By mouth:

powder	Pulver
powder mixtures	Pulvermischungen
granules	Granulat
effervescent granules	Brausegranulat
pills	Pillen
capsules	Kapseln
(hard gelatine capsules)	(Hartgelatinekapseln)
(soft gelatine capsules)	(Weichgelatinekapseln)
(retard capsules)	(Retardkapseln)
various teas	Teemischungen
instant tea	Pulvertee
tea bags	Teeaufgussbeutel
extract	Extrakt
tincture	Tinktur
suspension	Suspension
emulsion	Emulsion
tablets	Tabletten
effervescent tablets	Brausetabletten
coated tablets	Dragees
chewable tablets	Kautabletten
sublingual tablets (taken under the tongue)	Sublingualtabletten
solution	Lösung
drops	Tropfen
juice	(Frucht-)Saft
syrup	Sirup
homeopathic solutions	homöopathische Lösungen
dilutions	Dilutionen
gargle	Gurgellösung
washing solution	Spüllösung

External application:

paste	Paste
ointment	Salbe
cream	Creme
gel	Gel
greasy ointment	Fettsalbe
solution	Lösung
spray	Spray
powder	Puder
emulsion	Emulsion
lotion	Lotion
tincture	Tinktur
liniment	Liniment
balsam	Balsam
plaster	Pflaster

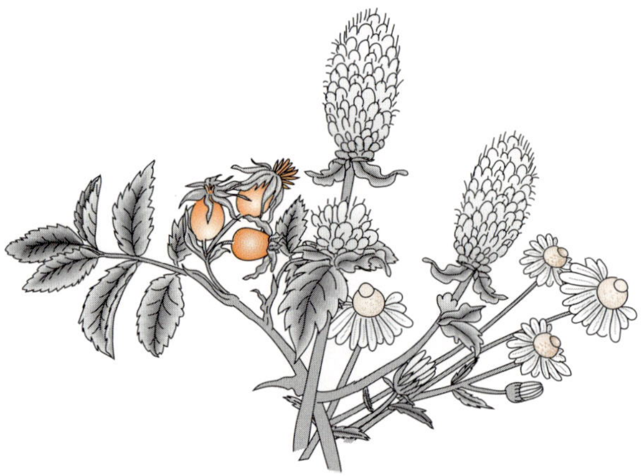

Parenteral administration (by injection):

infusion (aqueous solution)	Infusionslösung
injection	Injektionslösung
ampules	Ampullen
vial	Injektionsflaschen

Eye administration:

eyedrops	Augentropfen
(aqueous eyedrops)	(wässrige Augentropfen)
(lubricant eyedrops)	(ölige Augentropfen)
eye ointment	Augensalbe
eye solution	Augenbad

Ear administration:

eardrops	Ohrentropfen

Intranasal application (up the nose):

nose drops	Nasentropfen
nose ointment	Nasensalbe
nose spray	Nasenspray
nose gel	Nasengel

For inhalation:

aerosol	Dosier-Aerosol
for inhalation	Inhalationslösung

Drugs for vaginal administration:

vaginal cream	Vaginalcreme
vaginal suppositories	Vaginalzäpfchen

By rectum:

suppositories	Suppositorien = Zäpfchen
ointment, cream (rectal ointment)	Salbe, Creme (Rektal-Salbe)
combination pack: ointment and suppositories	Kombipackung = Salbe + Zäpfchen
enema	Klysma = Einlauf = Klistier

3.3. Herbs and spices

aconite	Eisenhut
anise	Anis
arnica	Arnika
birch	Birke
blackberry	Brombeere
blueberry	Heidelbeere
broom	Ginster
camomile	Kamille
caraway	Kümmel
cardamom	Kardamom
cherry	Kirsche
cinnamon	Zimt
club-moss	Bärlapp
coltsfoot	Huflattich
cornflower	Kornblume
cowslip	Schlüsselblume, Primel
dandelion	Löwenzahn
deadly nightshade	Tollkirsche, Belladonna
deadnettle	Taubnessel
elder	Holunder
eucalyptus	Eucalyptus
fennel	Fenchel
gentian	Enzian
ginger	Ingwer
hawthorn	Weißdorn
hemp	Hanf
hop	Hopfen
horse chestnut	Rosskastanie
horsetail	Schachtelhalm, Zinnkraut
ipecac	Brechwurzel, Ipecacuanha
iris	Schwertlilie
ivy	Efeu
juniper	Wacholder
laurel	Lorbeer
lavender	Lavendel
lemon tree	Zitronenbaum
lily of the valley	Maiglöckchen
lime tree	Linde
linseed	Leinsamen
liquorice root	Süßholzwurzel
lovage	Liebstöckl
majoram	Majoran
mallow	Malve
marigold	Ringelblume
marshmallow	Eibisch
meadow saffron	Herbstzeitlose
melissa	Melisse
mistletoe	Mistel
mugwort	Beifuß
myrrh	Myrrhe
nutmeg	Muskatnuss
onion	Zwiebel
pepper	Pfeffer
plantain	Wegerich
poppy	Mohn
potato	Kartoffel
raspberry	Himbeere
rhubarb	Rhabarber
rice	Reis
rose	Rose
rose-hip	Hagebutte
rosemary	Rosmarin
rye	Roggen
saffron	Safran, Crocus
sage	Salbei
seaweed	Tang
senna	Senna
stinging nettle	Brennessel
strawberry	Erdbeere
thyme	Thymian
tumeric	Gelbwurz
valerian	Baldrian
walnut	Walnuss
wheat	Weizen
willow	Weide
woodruff	Waldmeister
wormwood	Wermut
yarrow	Schafgarbe

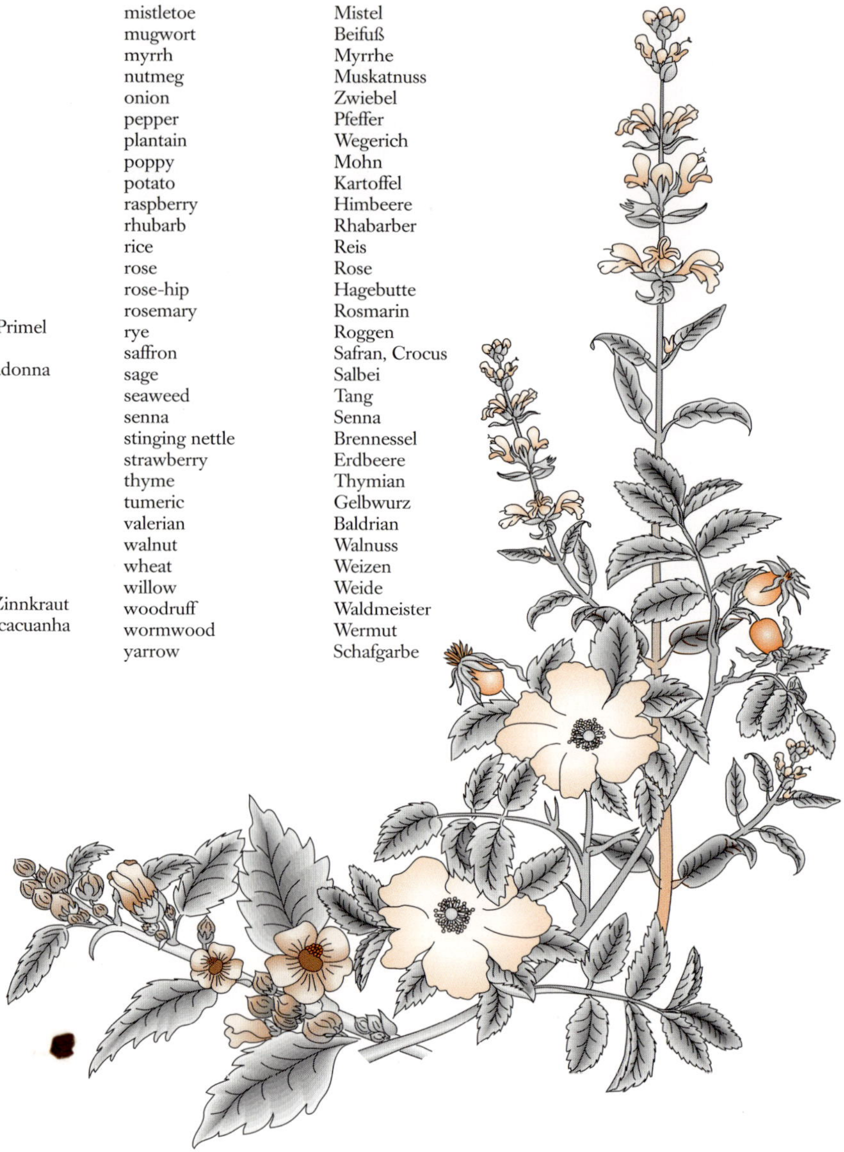

3.4. Baby care

Mrs Potter is pregnant. She is having her first baby and wants to prepare for it in good time. This is her shopping list for the chemist's:

baby scales
napkins
tissues
baby cream
baby lotion
baby powder
cotton swabs
bath thermometer
sterilizing tablets
feeding bottles
bottle warmer
teats
formula
dummies
baby bath
baby shampoo
tea
blunt-ended scissors for nails *3
lactose

Mrs Mark's son, Mike, is nine months old. She stopped breast-feeding some weeks ago and now gives him all kinds of baby food, which she usually buys in jars at the chemist's. They might contain:

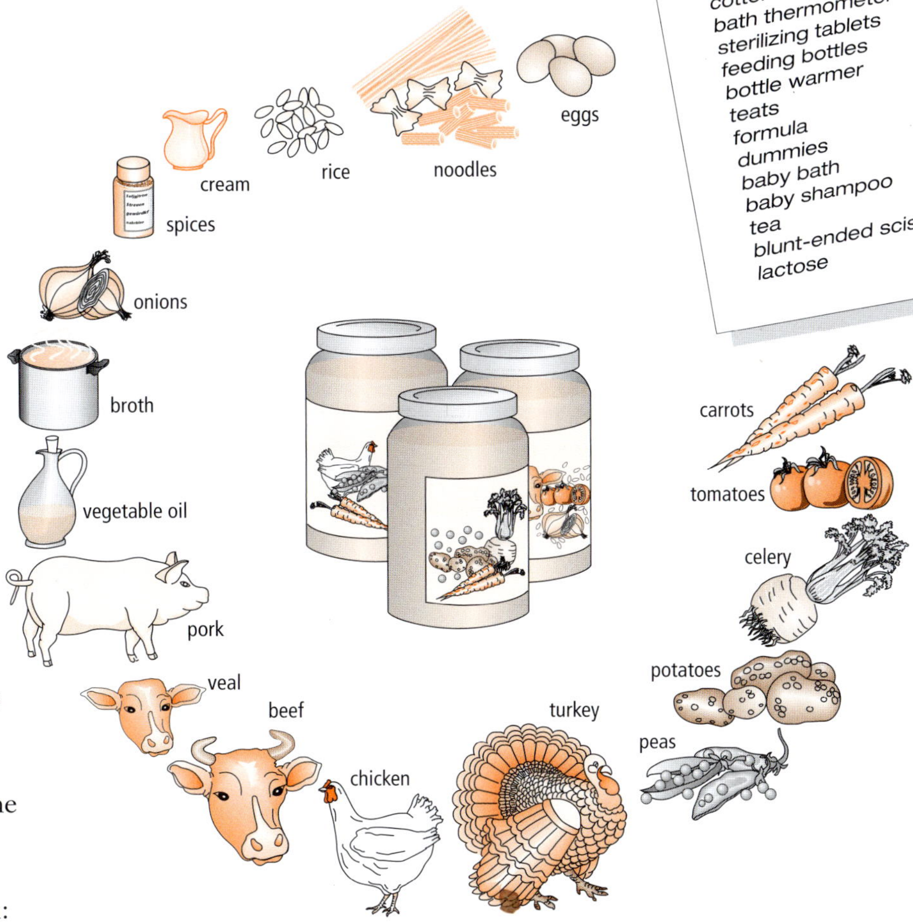

*3) 'Nappy' is the abbreviation for 'napkin'; in American English it is called 'diaper'. 'Cotton swabs' are sometimes called 'cotton-tipped sticks' or 'cotton buds'. The American word for 'teat' is 'nipple'. 'Dummies' are 'called' 'pacifiers' in America.

When Mike is thirsty, he gets either tea or fruit juice:

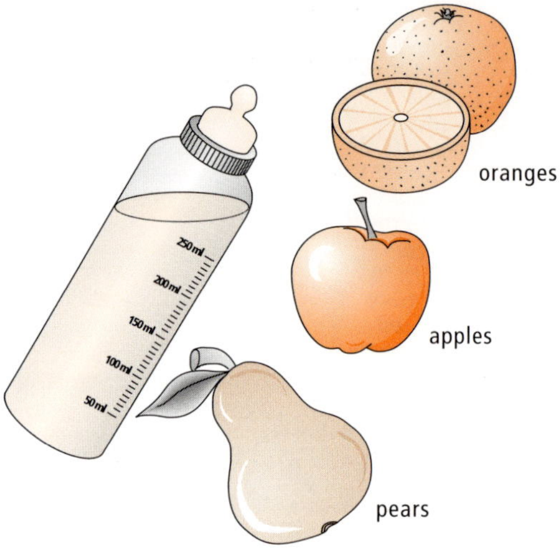

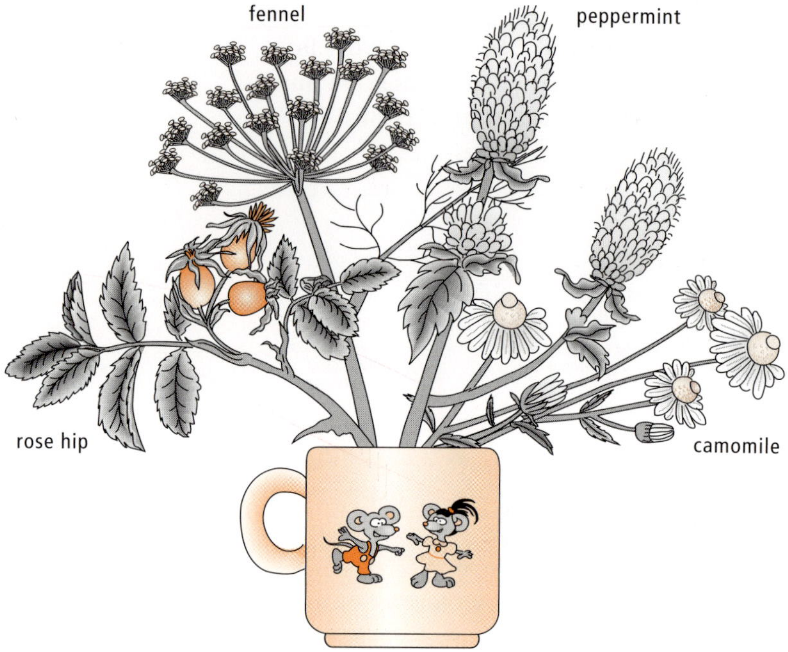

Fig. 3.4.: Fruit and herbs

In the evening Mike prefers to eat purees of apples, bananas or apricots, sometimes mixed with wholemeal cereals. The powdered baby food Mrs Mark buys contains oatmeal, wheat, corn, semolina, rice, cornflakes, powdered milk, nuts, honey and lots of vitamins and mineral substances. They are essential in a healthy diet and are especially important for a growing child. It is very easy to prepare Mike's porridge. Mrs Mark just has to add boiled water or milk to the powder and stir it – then it is ready to serve.

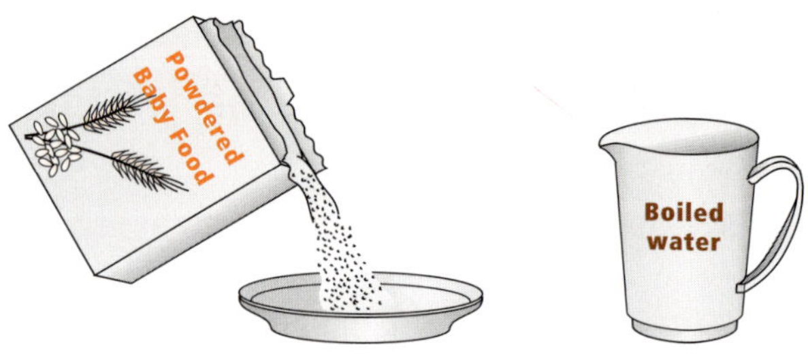

3.5. First aid

Accidents are a major cause of death in all modern societies. Each year 20–70 people per 100,000 inhabitants die in accidents. Young people, in particular, are much more likely to suffer accidental death than to die from a serious disease. By far the most important causes of accidental death are motor vehicle accidents, which account for about fifty percent of such deaths. Home accidents, as well, claim a large number of victims every year, in particular among old people and small children.

Everybody should have a knowledge of basic first aid and every home, car, boat or rucksack should contain a first aid kit, which must be accessible, in a portable box, unlocked – but out of children's reach. All medicines should be clearly labelled and dressings well wrapped.

All items for a first aid kit can be bought at the chemist's:

*4) There are various kinds of bandage, e.g. 'gauze bandage', 'crepe bandage', 'elastic bandage'. You can say 'sticking plaster' or 'elastoplast' or 'bandaid'. An 'adhesive strapping' can also be called 'first aid tape'.

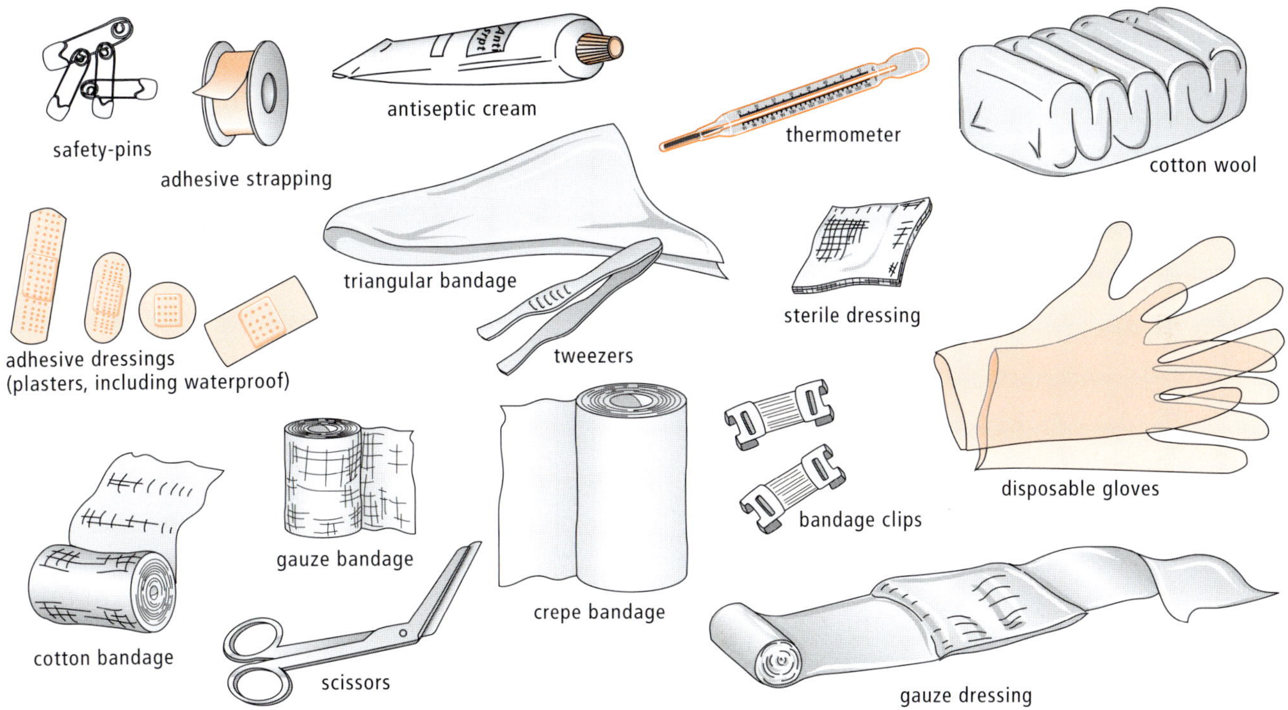

Fig. 3.5.: First aid kit (*4)

3.6. Beauty care and personal hygiene

A lot of people buy items at the chemist's for beauty care and personal hygiene. They expect to receive high quality products and better advice than in an ordinary shop.

Have a look at the following advertisements:

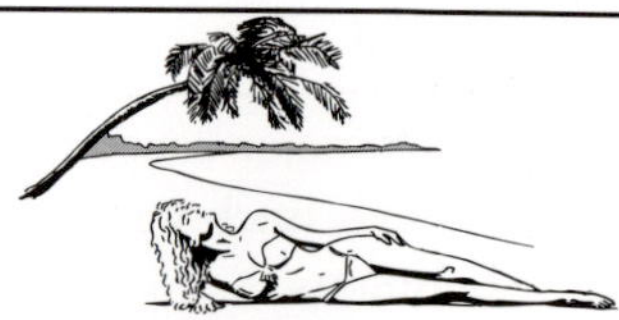

Sole sun care ABC

A Don't sunbathe for longer than 15 minutes on your first day on the beach. Then you can gradually increase it.

B Never lie for more than 30 minutes at a time in the sun. Move around or go for a swim.

C Re-apply your suntan cream after swimming.

D Never fall asleep in the sun.

E Avoid the midday sun.

F Stay out of the sun at the first sign of any skin irritation until the soreness disappears.

G Drink plenty of water or fruit juice when you are sunbathing to ensure sufficient moisture intake.

H Immediately put moisturizer on your face and use body lotion after sunbathing.

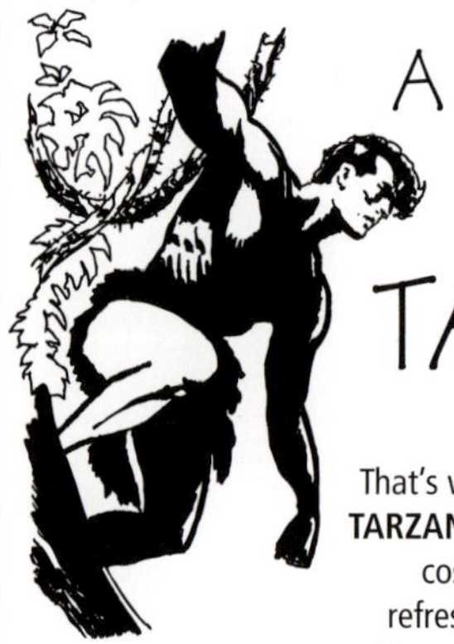

A MAN IS A WINNER WITH TARZAN

That's what women like about men: **TARZAN**, a remarkable line of men's cosmetics. Masculine fragrance refreshes the skin. A bold scent of its own, without being unpleasant

Pre-shave lotion
Ideal preparation for an electric shave.

After-shave cream
TARZAN'S own idea for soothing, better skin care. Skin cream blended with after shave lotion. Highly effective with its 53% pure alcohol.

Deodorant stick
TARZAN deodorant stops body odour immediately, effectively. All day long.

Sweet breath throughout the day

DENTY MOUTHWASH
Put some drops of DENTY MOUTHWASH into a glass every morning. Then fill the glass up with water and rinse your mouth and throat. This will keep your breath sweet throughout the day.

DENTY TOOTHPASTE
perfects the care of the mouth. Refreshing and pleasantly flavoured. DENTY TOOTHPASTE contains essential ingredients to take care of your teeth.

DENTY TOOTHBRUSHES
guarantee perfect care of the teeth and the gums. You can reach all parts of the mouth with this toothbrush. It has been produced in accordance with the latest scientific research.

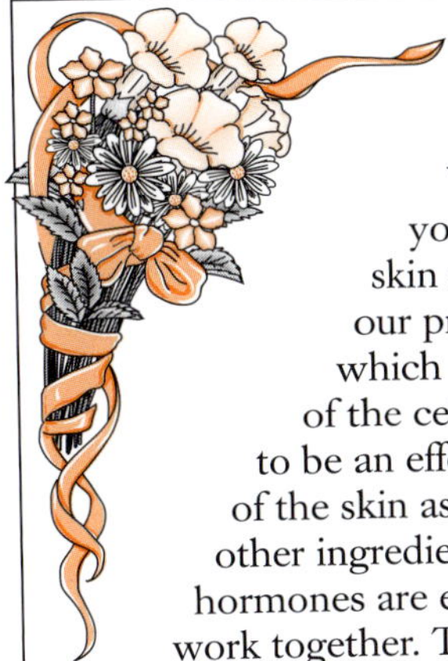

Beauty advice

Dear Madam,
We congratulate you on your decision to give your skin active beauty treatment. All our products contain Allantoin, which promotes the regeneration of the cells. Furthermore it is known to be an effective cure for irritation of the skin as well as abrasions. All other ingredients such as vitamins and hormones are especially formulated to work together. This is what your skin needs besides moisture and oil to remain young and elastic.

We recommend using small quantities as our products contain sufficient amounts of all ingredients to provide essential daily protection.

Every morning your skin needs cleansing, firming, protecting.

Every evening your skin needs cleansing, firming, nourishing.

Cleansing milk
Cleanses your skin thouroughly and gently removes dust, make-up and impurities without affecting the proper chemical balance of the skin.
Instructions for use: Apply to face and neck in the morning as well as in the evening. Leave for a few minutes and remove with tissue or cotton wool. Moisturize and firm with face lotion.

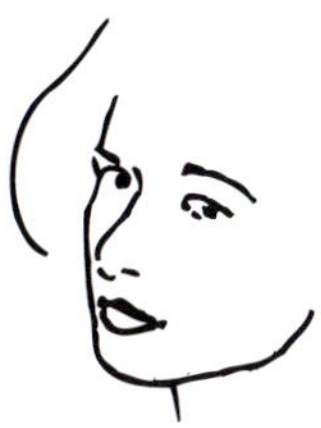

Face lotion
Moisturizes and firms your skin. Renders dry skin more resistant and works against impurities.
Instructions for use: Add a small quantity to cotton wool and apply to face after cleansing each morning and evening. For normal and dry skin apply facial lotion on a moist piece of cotton wool.

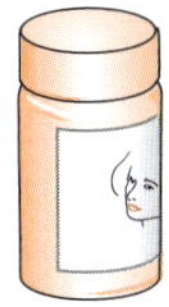

Regenerating cream for mature skin
This cream is enriched with regenerating emollients, hormones and other special ingredients that stimulate regeneration. It returns the youthful look to your skin and prevents wrinkles.
Instructions for use: Each evening after cleansing and conditioning apply gently to face and throat. Massage starting at the base of throat and working upwards.

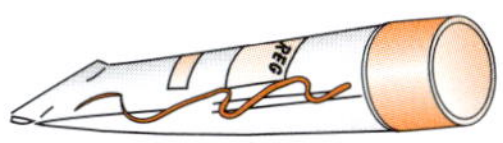

Day cream
This transparent cream is formulated with moisturizing ingredients to protect your skin against impurities. At the same time it provides an ideal make-up base.
Instructions for use: Smooth on face and throat daily after cleansing and conditioning and massage gently.

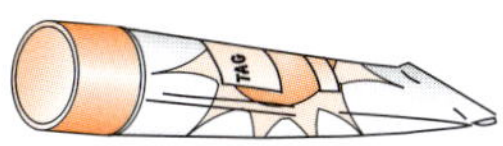

Night cream
A rich cream that is absorbed instantly by your skin and provides constant nourishing of the skin texture. The natural ingredients stimulate the circulation and leave your skin radiant and young.
Instructions for use:
Use in the evening after cleansing and conditioning. Apply to face and throat with fingertips and massage gently.

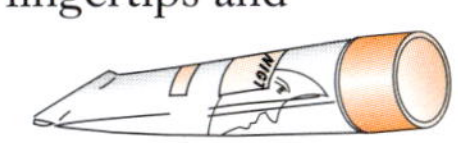

✳ Übungen zu Kapitel 3 ab Seite 54.

Good morning, can I help you?

Guten Morgen, kann ich Ihnen helfen?

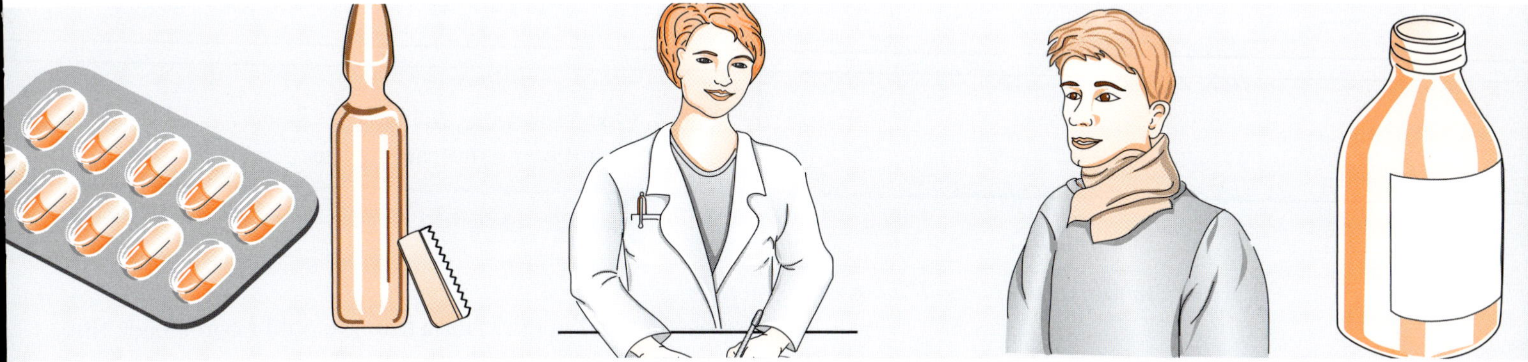

4.1. Conversation at the chemist's

Part one

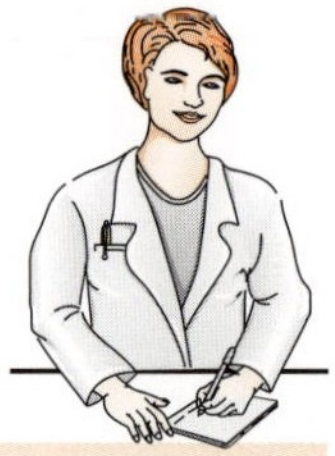

Chemist

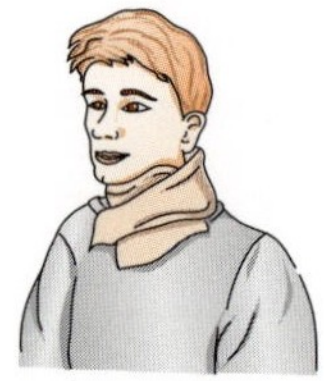

Customer

Good morning, sir,
What can I do for you?

Good morning, madam.
I want some ointment, please.

Do you have a prescription?

Yes, I do. Here it is.

Would you take a seat, please. It'll take a few minutes.

Oh, I'm in rather a hurry. Could I come back this afternoon?

Yes, what about four o'clock?

Can't you manage it before?

Alright, at two.

Oh, I almost forgot, I need some cotton wool and a bandage.

How wide do you want the bandage?

10 cm, please. And a bottle of Sana face lotion.

Here you are.

Thank you.

Is there anything else I can do for you?

No thank you. That's all.
How much is it?

It's € 8.90 (eight euro ninety).

Here you are. I'll come back for my prescription at two.

It should be ready by then.

Goodbye.

Bye-bye.

4.1.1. Beginning of a conversation

(Expressions marked with * or + can be used alternatively as their meaning is almost the same)

Man begrüßt sich:

Good morning, madam (sir)
Mr Miller (Mrs ..., Miss ...)
Good afternoon, ...
Good evening, ...
*Hello, ...
*Hi, ... (*1)

Nun fragt die Apothekerin/der Apotheker:

*What can I do for you?
*Can (May) I help you?
+ Are you next?
+ Who's next?
+ Next, please.

4.1.2. The customer's problems and requests

*I would like ...
*I want ...
*I need ...
*Please, give me ...
*A (some) ..., please.
*Have you got ...?
*Can I have ...?
*Could you give me ...?
*Do you have ...?
*Do you sell ...?
Have you got a book on ...?

Und der Kunde äußert seine Wünsche:
Er hat (k)ein Rezept:

*My doctor gave me this prescription.
*My doctor has prescribed ...
Can you make up this prescription for me, please.
Do I need a prescription for ...?

Der Kunde beschreibt seine Beschwerden:

*Have you got a remedy for ...?
*Can you recommend something for ...?
I've got pains in my ...
I'm feeling a little weak in my legs, but it's better today.
I'm feeling the weather. Can you give me something for my blood circulation (rheumatism, ...)?

*1) 'Hello' can also be spelled 'hallo' or 'hullo'. It is more colloquial than 'good morning'. 'Hi' is used more by Americans.

4.1.3. The chemist's questions and comments

Hat der Kunde ein (korrektes) Rezept?

*Do you have a prescription?
*Have you got a prescription?
You need a (German, new) prescription for this medicine.
Ask your doctor to write a prescription for this medicine.

Die Apothekerin/der Apotheker muss das Alter des Patienten wissen:

How old is the patient?

Sie/Er schickt den Kunden erst einmal zum Arzt:

*Did you consult a doctor? (*2)
*It would be better to consult a doctor (a specialist).
* ... to go to a doctor.
* ... to see a doctor.
It's necessary (for you) to consult a ...

Und sie/er beschreibt den Weg dorthin:

The nearest doctor (dentist, oculist ...) is in Church Street. Go down (along) Park Street, cross Manchester Square, turn left (right) into Church Street. Dr Smith's practice is in the second building opposite the station on the first floor.

Die Apothekerin/der Apotheker braucht noch ein paar Informationen:

Do you have a health insurance?
*Where are you employed?
*Which firm do you work for?
You must send this certificate to your health insurance.

Das Arzneimittel muss hergestellt werden:

Your medicine will have to be made up.
Would you take a seat, please, for a few minutes.(*3)
Your medicine will be ready in a few minutes.
... this afternoon.
(evening)
... in half an hour.

*2) In English you never 'visit' a doctor unless you have tea with him.

*3) Speak politely to the customer:
You can say:
'Sit down for a few minutes, please.'
But it is more polite to say:
'Would you (could you) – But this is very formal.) sit down for a few minutes, please.'
Or: 'Would you be so kind as to sit down for a few minutes, please.'
But this is very formal.

Ein Arzneimittel muss bestellt werden:

I'll have to order your medicine.
Could you come back later, please,
... in an hour.
... this afternoon (evening).
... tomorrow morning.
... on Monday (Tuesday) (*4) morning.
... in three days.

Die Öffnungszeiten der Apotheke:

Our pharmacy (chemist's shop, dispensary) (*5) is open from 8 a.m. till (to) 6 p.m. (*6)
Our pharmacy is closed from ...
Our pharmacy is open the whole day.
We are open late (all night), you can come after 6 p.m.
... , it doesn't matter if you come late.

4.1.4. Other useful terms for a conversation at the chemist's

Der Kunde ist wohl Ausländer:

Where do you come from?
Are you English (American, Australian, Japanese ...)?

Deshalb hat die Apothekerin/der Apotheker Probleme, ihn zu verstehen:

Pardon (Sorry), I didn't understand.
Could you speak a little more slowly, please.

Do you speak German (English, ...)?

Ein häufiges Thema: Das Wetter

What a nice (wonderful, hot, cool, ...) day today, isn't it?

Und die Frage nach dem Befinden:

How are you, Mr (Mrs, Miss) ...?
How is your husband (wife, daughter, son, mother, father, ...)?
Are you (is she, he) feeling better today?
I'm sorry to hear you haven't been well.
Do you have a temperature?
Is your stomach (throat, arm, foot) alright again?
You must take care of yourself. You look very pale.
I hope you'll feel better soon.

*4) The days of the week are always written with a capital letter: Monday, Tuesday, Wednesday, Thursday, Friday, Saturday, Sunday

*5) Americans usually say 'drugstore' instead of chemist's (shop), pharmacy or dispensary. The people working there are called chemist, pharmacist, dispenser.

*6) 'a.m.' (ante meridiem) is used for the time from midnight till noon, 'p.m.' (post meridiem) is used for the time after noon.

4.1.5. End of the conversation

Die Apothekerin/der Apotheker übergibt die Ware:

Here you are.
Thank you very much.
*Will that be all?
*Is there anything else I can do for you?
Do you want a plastic bag?

Nichts ist umsonst:

*How much is it?
*How much do I owe you?
*What does it cost?
+It is ...
+It costs ...
You have to pay ...

Ein paar gute Wünsche zum Schluss:

I wish you a speedy recovery.
Have a good journey.
Have a nice holiday.
Have a nice weekend.
Good luck.
Best wishes (*7) to your husband (wife, ...).

*7) It's better to say 'Remember me to your (husband)' if you don't know the person well.

Und auf Wiedersehen:

*Goodbye.
*Bye-bye.

4.2. Conversation at the chemist's

Part two

Chemist

Customer

Hello, Mary. I haven't seen you for ages.

Good morning, Mr Miller. We've just come back from Italy.

Did you have a nice holiday there?

It was lovely. But on our way home Mother caught a bad cold.

Did she consult a doctor?

Yes, Dr Smith came this morning and prescribed something for it. Here's the prescription.

Let's see. So you take these tablets for the fever and this syrup for the cough.

Can you explain how the medicine is to be taken.

Of course, dear. Your mother has to take two tablets in the morning, two at noon and two in the evening.

Does she have to take the tablets before or after meals?

Preferably before meals.

And the cough mixture?

She should take one tablespoonful every four hours. If you can't remember all this, it's written on the label.

Thank you, Mr Miller. How much do I owe you?

You have to pay € 10 (ten euro), please.

Here you are.

Thank you, Mary. Bye-bye and give my regards to your mother.

Goodbye, Mr Miller.

*8) 'Children' is the irregular plural of 'child' (compare: man – men, woman – women, foot – feet). The possessive cases of these nouns are formed as follows: the man's legs the men's legs (compare: the boy's legs – the boys' legs)

4.2.1. General instructions

Die Aufbewahrung des Medikaments:

This medicine should be kept tightly closed.
* Keep this medicine away from light.
* ... out of direct sunlight.
+ Keep this medicine out of children's (*8) reach.
+ ... out of reach of children.
This medicine must be kept in a cool place.
Keep your medicine in the fridge (= refrigerator), but not in the deepfreezer.
Warning: This medicine is highly inflammable.

Vorsicht, nicht einnehmen:

This medicine is for external use only.
* It must not be taken.
* Not to be taken.
This medicine is toxic if inhaled or swallowed.
* Keep this medicine away from your eyes (mucous membranes ...).
* Avoid contact with eyes (mucous membranes ...).
Danger: Poison!

Dieses Arzneimittel muss eingenommen werden, aber in Maßen:

Do you know how to take the medicine?
The dose may be repeated four times a day, if required.
It is dangerous to exceed the recommended dose.

Und so steht es auf dem Beipackzettel:

Dosage: In the absence of specific instructions from your doctor this medicine should be taken (applied) as follows:
Children under 1 year
Children 1 to 7 years: ...

4.2.2. Specific instructions for use

4.2.2.1. Tablets (pills), capsules

Wie viele Tabletten soll der Patient nehmen?

Take	one tablet	a day (a week)
	... half a tablet	a day ...
	... three tablets	a day ...

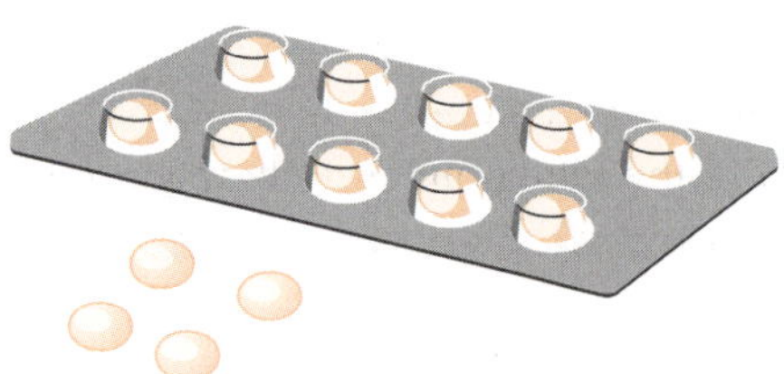

Und wann soll er sie nehmen?

Take one tablet in the morning
... at noon.
... in the evening.
... at night.
... every hour (= hourly).
... every three hours.
... every day (morning, evening).

Vor oder nach dem Essen, mit oder ohne Flüssigkeit?

*Take one tablet (preferably)
* ... before breakfast.
... before meals.
... with your meals.
... after meals.
... with water (if required, if desired, if necessary).
... with tea.
... with liquid.

Sollen die Tabletten geschluckt, aufgelöst oder gelutscht werden?

This tablet should not be chewed.
It should be swallowed whole.

Dissolve in water.
... in liquid.

Suck one tablet slowly every two hours.
Let the tablet melt slowly in your mouth.
Put the tablet under your tongue.

4.2.2.2. Drops, syrups, mixtures, solutions

Vor Gebrauch schütteln!

*Shake the bottle well before taking the drops (syrup).
* ... you take the drops.
This mixture can be taken undiluted.

Wann und wie sollen die Tropfen eingenommen werden?

Take 15 drops before breakfast and at bedtime.
... on a lump of sugar (honey).
... in half a cup of hot water.
... with liquid.
... undiluted.
... in a tablespoonful of cold water.
Put 20 drops into a glass of hot water and rinse your mouth (throat).

Der Packung liegt ein Messlöffel bei:

Take one (two, three) measuring spoonful(s).

Es gibt Augentropfen:

Put one drop in each eye three times a day.
... in your right (left) eye.
... in the sore (inflamed) eye.
Once opened the eyedrops should be used within 4 weeks.

Und Nasentropfen:

Apply three drops in the nose.
... in the right (left) nostril.
... in the sore (inflamed) nostril.

Tropfen gegen Hühneraugen:

Apply one drop on the corn.

Lösungen zum Gurgeln:

To gargle dilute the solution with warm water.

Und Zusätze für das Badewasser:

This remedy has to be added to bath water.
Use three measuring spoonfuls
...for a complete bath.
...for a hip bath.

4.2.2.3. Suppositories

Wie viele Zäpfchen?

Insert one suppository daily.
Insert two suppositories daily into the anus.

Wann soll man sie einführen?

Insert one suppository as required.
Insert whenever an attack of fever occurs, ...

Und so steht es auf dem Beipackzettel:

Remove wrapping and insert ...
Insert as prescribed by the doctor ...

4.2.2.4. Creams, ointments, gels

Wie ist die Salbe aufzutragen?

Apply the ointment thickly (thinly).
... three times a day.
Rub it into your skin.
Don't rub it in.
Cover the wound with ointment.

Was geschieht dann?

*Dress the wound.
*Apply a bandage.
Leave the wound open.

Vorsicht bei manchen Salben!

Wash your hands after applying the ointment.
*Avoid contact with the eyes.
*Keep away from ...

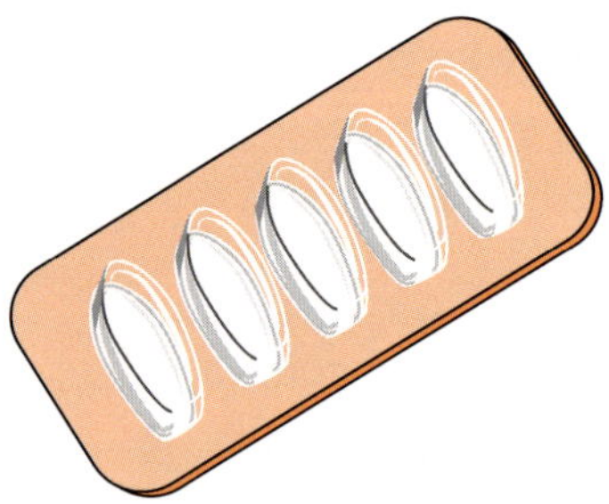

4.2.2.5. Powders (*9)

Puder kann äußerlich angewendet werden:

Take a minute quantity of powder and ...
Sprinkle the powder on the wound.
... on the skin.

Und Pulver innerlich:

Put one teaspoonful in a cup of hot water.
Take half a tablespoonful in ...
Put the contents in half a cup of warm water and sip it slowly.
Dissolve three teaspoonfuls in a cup of water and ...
Mix with half a glass of cold water.

4.2.2.6. Teas

Zur Aufbewahrung des Tees ist zu sagen:

This tea must be kept tightly closed.

Und so kann er zubereitet werden:

Boil the water.
Steep for 5 minutes.
Make the tea with cold water.
Dissolve 1 teaspoonful of instant tea in a cup of hot water.

⁎ Übungen zu Kapitel 4 ab Seite 57

4.2.2.7. Ampules

Den Inhalt von Ampullen kann man injizieren:

Take these ampules to your doctor, please.

Oder trinken:

Use the enclosed saw to open the ampule and drink it undiluted.

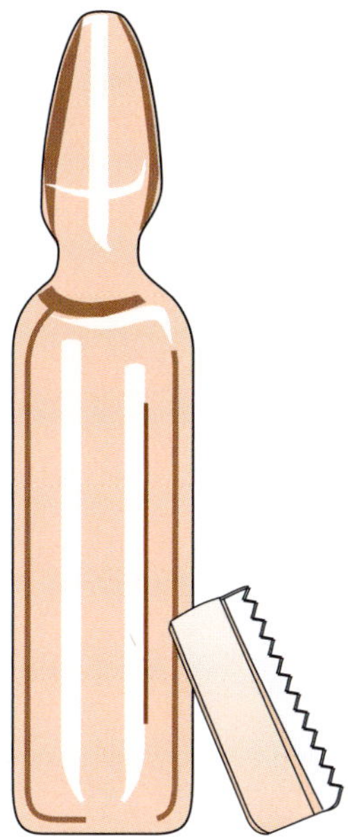

*9) The German translation for 'powder' can be 'Puder' oder 'Pulver'.

Exercises | Übungen

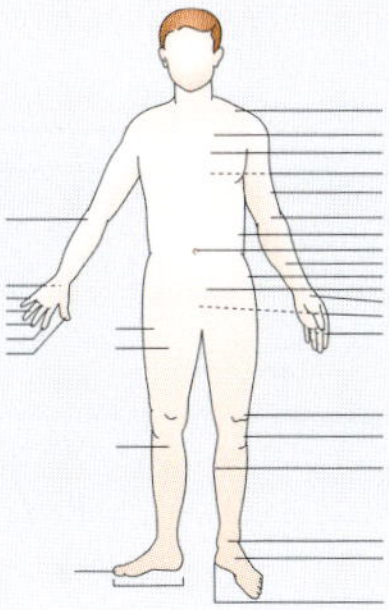

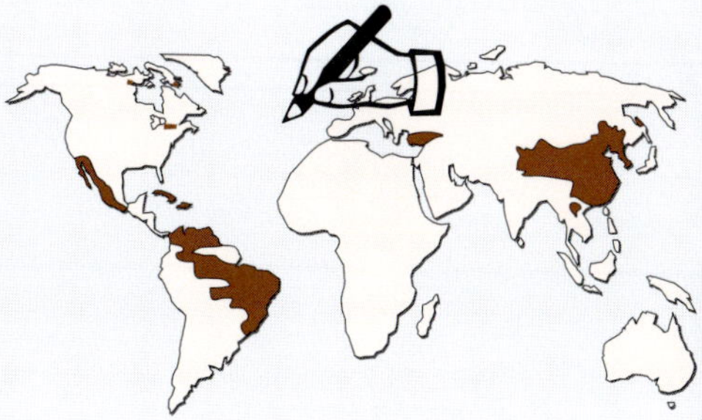

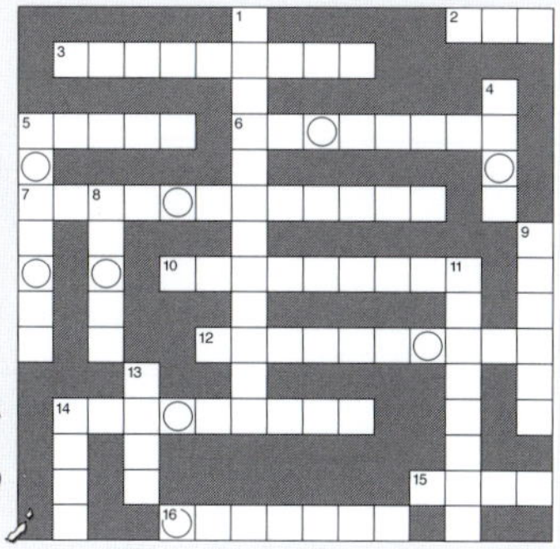

5

5.1. Exercises chapter one

1. Label the diagram, please.

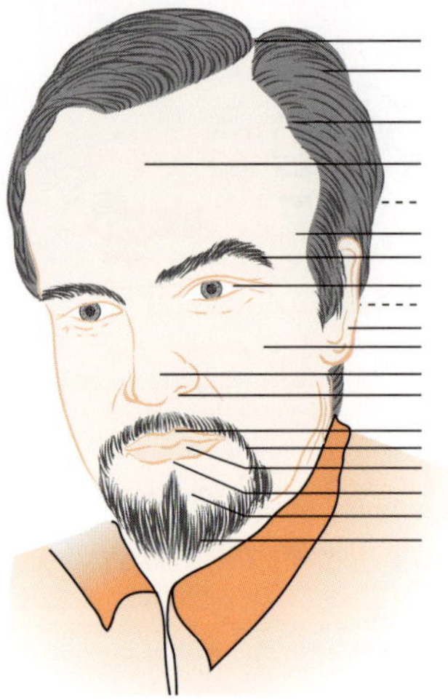

2. Which parts of the body can you remember?

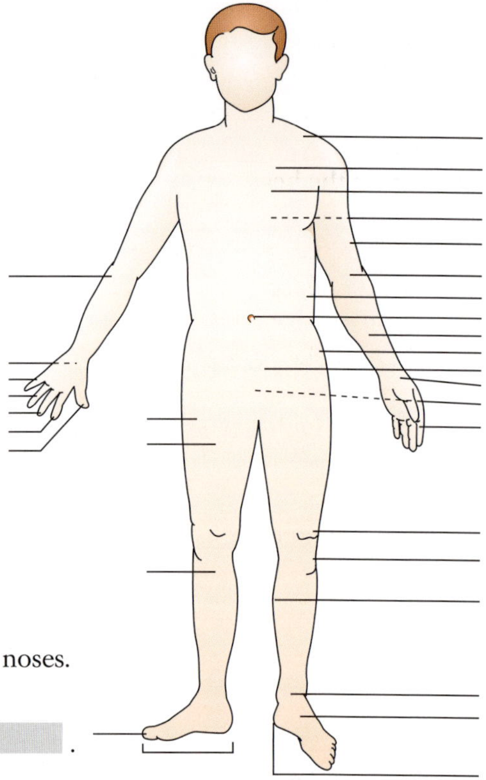

3. Can you answer the following questions?

a) The largest gland in the body is the ________.

b) ________ are those little brown spots some people get in the summer on their cheeks and noses.

c) All long bones contain ________.

d) Other terms for backbone are ________ and ________.

e) Most people get their first ________ round the eyes.

f) The bones of the forearm are called the ________ and the ________.

g) The ________, which helps to make the blood pure, is situated to the left of the stomach.

h) The blood is transported from the heart to all parts of the body in the ________; it travels back to the heart in the ________.

i) ________ has the same meaning as sinew.

j) The ________ is stored in the gall bladder.

4. Crossword puzzle:

Across
1 part of the foot
3 the intestines
4 It's between the trunk and the head.
6 Many people nowadays have problems with their ...
9 part of the head
12 part of the mouth
13 part of the inside of the mouth
15 part of the leg
16 the upper part of the trunk
17 We have five of them on each foot.
18 It's on our head.
20 It's the joint between the upper arm and the forearm.
21 another term for bile
22 A man who is not clean-shaven grows a ...
23 It's the entrance to our digestive system.
24 We have 16 teeth in each ...

Down
2 We need it to be able to see.
5 It is below the mouth.
7 It is enclosed by the breastbone and the ribs.
8 It's the bone inside the nose.
10 Little children call it 'belly'.
11 part of the hand
12 the plural of 12 across
14 part of the foot
16 the bone framework of the head
18 part of the trunk
19 = 17 Across
20 We need them to be able to hear.
21 It covers the base of each tooth.

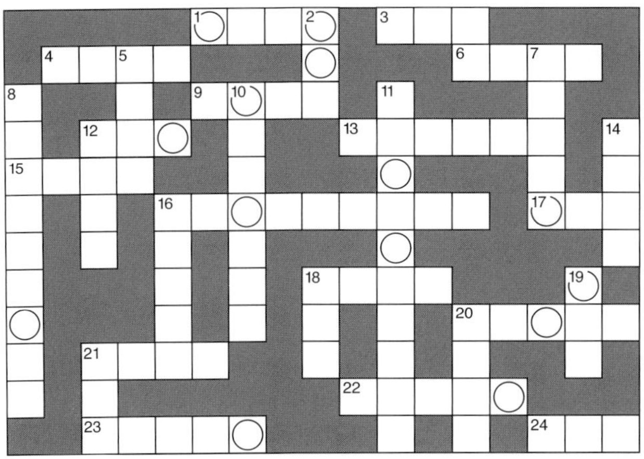

And now put the circled letters in the correct order:

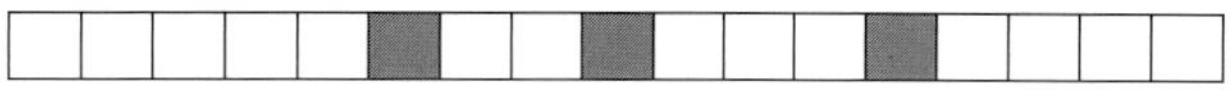

5.2. Exercises chapter two

1. Complete these sentences, please.

a) ______ is inflammation of the tonsils.
b) ______ is inflammation of the lungs.
c) ______ is inflammation of the sinuses.
d) ______ is inflammation of the bronchial tubes.
e) General signs of most colds are ______

2. Centrigrade and Fahrenheit:

a) Please convert the following temperatures from Centigrade into Fahrenheit:
25 °C, 40.3 °C
b) And now try to convert the following temperatures from Fahrenheit into Centrigrade:
80 °F, 100.7 °F

3. Can you answer these questions?

a) Which children's illnesses are accompanied by a rash?
b) Which other children's illnesses can you remember?
c) Have a look at the vaccination programme on p. 13. Do you know why it is particularly recommended that girls should be vaccinated against German measles?

4. Look at the information about cholera on p. 17 and try to answer the following questions:

a) Where do people who receive this information come from?
b) Which part of the body is affected when you have cholera?
c) What is the incubation period?
d) What are you supposed to do if you feel you might have cholera?
e) Which other tropical diseases are there (see fig. 2.11 on p. 17)?

5. Points for discussion:

The following map shows the average life expectancies in the world and the graph below gives some information about life expectancies in Europe in the past. Have a look at them and at the illustrations in Chapter 2 and discuss the questions:

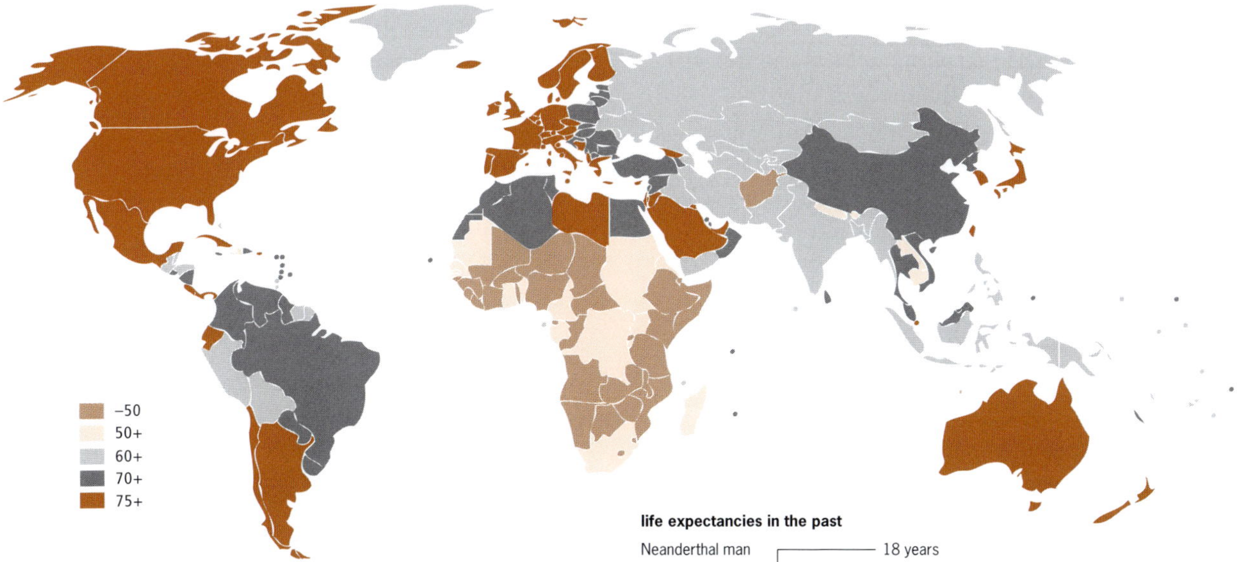

life expectancies in the past

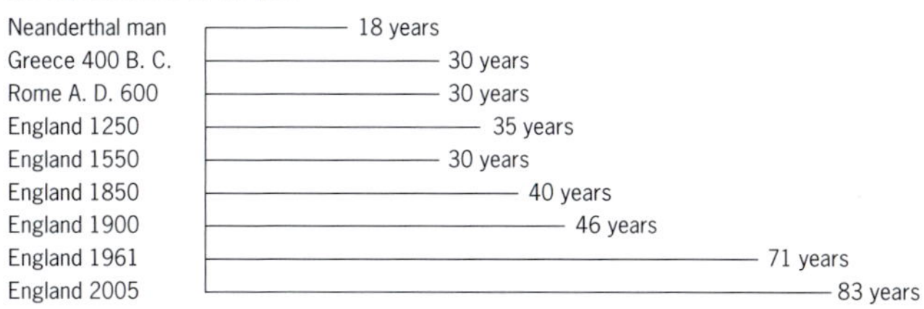

a) In which countries do people die rather young?
b) What might be the reasons?
c) Do people die from the same diseases all over the world?
d) What are the typical causes of death in Western Europe?
e) In which other parts of the world is the situation similar?
f) Can you give any explanation for this?
g) Which are the most important contributing factors to the risk of cardiac infarction?
h) Look at the graph on p. 14 and describe the frequency of cardiac infarctions in Germany during the last seventy years and try to give an explanation for this development.
i) The statistics on p. 15 show that far more people suffered from cancer in 2002 than at the beginning of the twentieth century. Which reason for this is given in the text?
j) Can you think of other reasons?
k) Was life expectancy in Europe always as high as it is today?
l) Which factors influenced life expectancy in the past?

6. Two crossword puzzles:

Across

2 the abbreviation for tuberculosis
3 inflammation of the lungs
5 a children's disease which affects the throat
6 pain in the back of the hip and thigh
7 inflammation of part of the large intestine
10 Someone with cholera suffers from it.
12 a children's disease which affects the throat, but fortunately has become very rare nowadays.
14 Some mushrooms might cause it.
15 If you suffer from sore throat, hoarseness, weariness, a runny nose and a cough, you might have caught ...
16 If you stay in the sun too long, you might suffer from ...

Down

1 the opposite of 10 across
4 another term for spots
5 a virus infection common in childhood
8 Nowadays children are vaccinated against this terrible disease.
9 Fortunately it's just a ..., not a fracture.
11 When you fall down and your skin gets scraped you have an ...
13 to vomit is to be ...
14 another word for ache

Put the circled letters in the correct order and finish the following sentence:

All these words are ...

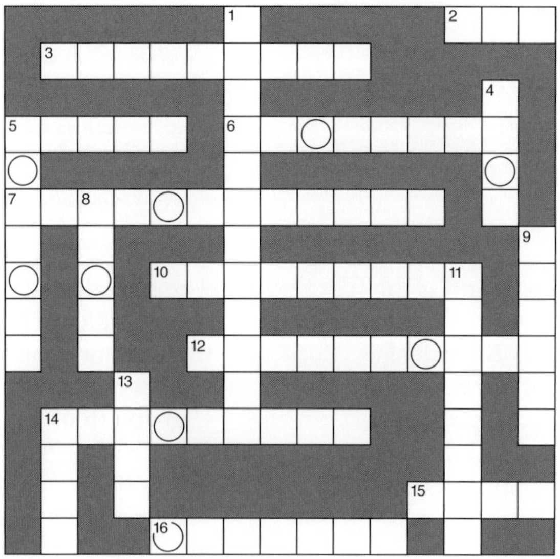

7. After you have answered 1–9 across, the second letter of each word forms another word:

1. enlarged mass of lymphoid tissue at the back of the nose
2. If someone's pancreas does not produce enough insulin he suffers from this disease.
3. to lose consciousness
4. painful contraction of a muscle often caused by cold or slight strain
5. If you break your arm, you've got a ...
6. a tropical disease
7. one of the signs of a cold; it might lead to bronchitis
8. a form of indigestion felt as a pain in the chest
9. a terrible disease, which can affect almost all organs of the body

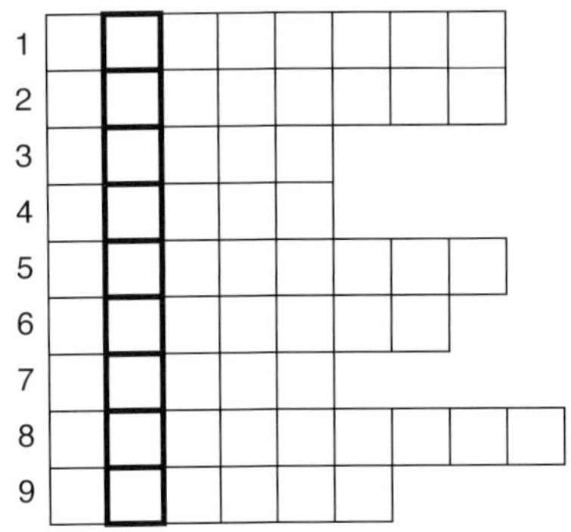

5.3. Exercises chapter three

1.

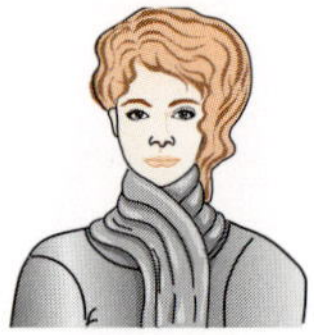

Jenny has a sore throat.

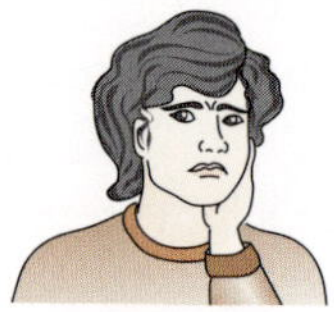

Brenda suffers from toothache.

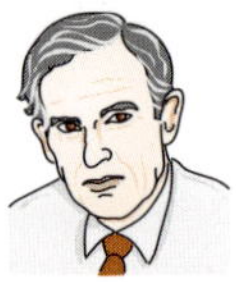

Tom has a headache and a temperature.

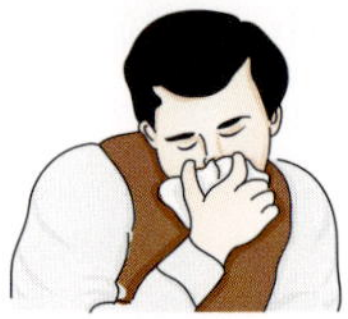

Jack sneezes all the time.

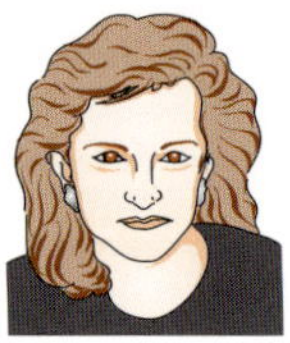

Mary can't sleep during the night because of her cough.

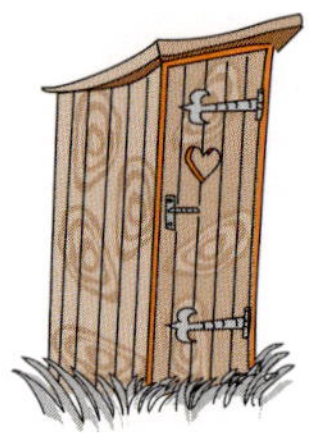

What has Peter got?

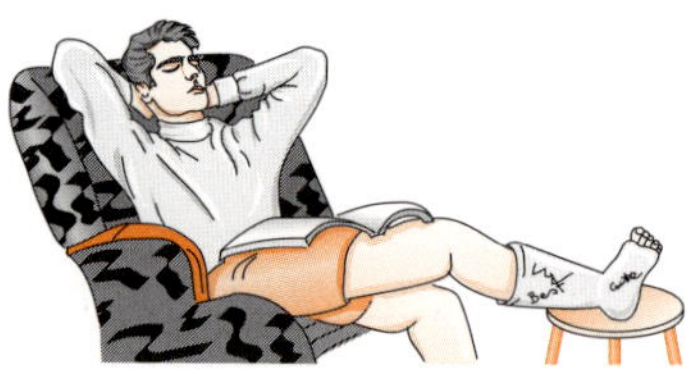

Bob has a swollen ankle.

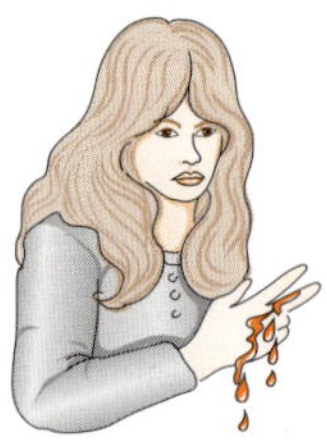

Jane has cut her finger.

They all go to the chemist's. What could they ask for to bring relief. Use the following expressions:

Have you got ...?
I need ...
Can I have ...?
Can you recommend ...?

2. Which items do you recognize?

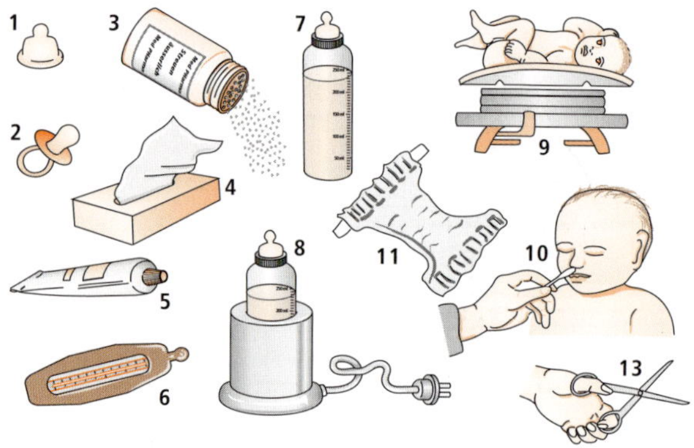

3. Can you complete the following clauses by those below?

1.) Although bandages and dressings can be improvised, b

2.) The first aider must avoid touching the wound or any part of the dressing d

3.) After applying a bandage, f

4.) The skin surrounding a wound should be clean and dry a

5.) If the injured person has an infection, c

6.) A sterile dressing should not be used e

a) before applying an adhesive plaster.
b) it is far better to have them on hand.
c) the first aider should wear disposable gloves.
d) which is in contact with the wound.
e) if the wrapping is damaged.
f) it is important to check that the circulation has not been affected.

4. Read the advertisements on pages 32 and 33, and try to answer the following questions:

TARZAN:
a) Can you explain the word “line”?
b) When does a man use pre-shave lotion and when does he use after-shave cream?
c) What are deodorants used for?

DENTY:
a) Can you explain how to use DENTY MOUTHWASH?
b) What are the characteristics of DENTY TOOTHPASTE?
c) What are toothbrushes supposed to be like?

Beauty advice:
a) What is the effect of Allantoin?
b) Which other ingredients do the products described contain?
c) What is said about the quantities that should be used?
d) What does the cleansing milk remove from your skin?
e) How are you supposed to apply face lotion?
f) What effects do day cream and night cream have on the skin?

5. Find out your hair type:

Fairy Hair Series
A series of especially selected hair groomers that really works for each hair type. Puts shine in dull, dry, bleached out hair. Cleans and fluffs out limp, lifeless, greasy hair.

1. Is your forehead
   A X dry
   B slightly greasy
   C quite greasy?
2. One day after shampooing does your scalp feel
   A itchy and tight
   B X comfortable
   C rather greasy?
3. How many days after shampooing does your hair lose its shine?
   A X It doesn’t. It improves after several days.

- **B** 2–4 days after shampooing
- **C** one day after shampooing.

4. Two days after shampooing is your hair
   - **A** just as good as or better than on the first day
   - **B** still holding up
   - **C** completely limp.
5. When you run a comb through your hair
   - **A** it seems coarse and brittle
   - **B** it presents no problem
   - **C** it seems thin.
6. Are broken or split ends
   - **A** a severe problem
   - **B** of moderate concern
   - **C** a slight problem?
7. Is your hair when wet
   - **A** tangled due to overbleaching or permanent wave
   - **B** difficult to comb
   - **C** relatively easy to comb?
8. In your regular hair care routine do you use hair dryers, curling pins, electric rollers
   - **A** once a week
   - **B** 2–4 times a week
   - **C** daily?
9. What would you most like a shampoo to do for your hair (besides washing it)
   - **A** have built-in conditioner for extreme dryness
   - **B** be mild enough to use often
   - **C** delay greasiness.

5 or more A's:
You have dry, brittle hair. Use series I.

5 or more B's or a combination of A's and B's or B's and C's:
Your hair is normal. Series II ist best for you.

5 or more C's:
Series III is best for greasy and limp hair.

6. A puzzle:

Answer 1–6 across and then read down the second letter of each word. This should form a word that means freedom from disease.

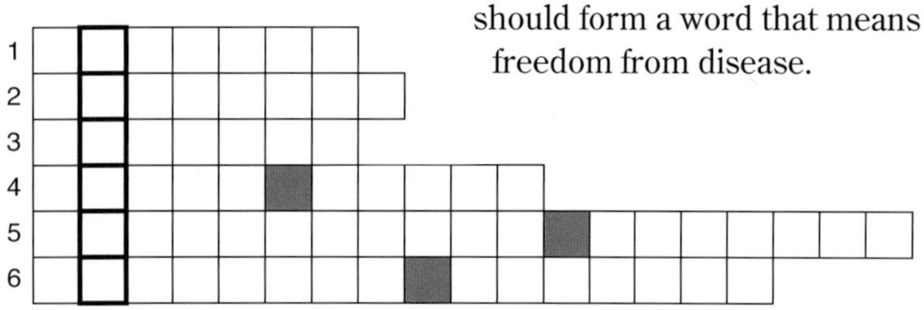

1.) You wash your hair with it.
2.) Some people take it when they are in pain or suffer from insomnia.
3.) Babies are sometimes given it when they suffer from constipation.
4.) What should scissors for babies' nails be like?
5.) You can use them for cleaning babies' bottles, teats and dummies.
6.) Someone who suffers from diarrhoea will take them.

5.4. Exercises chapter four

Part one

1. Fill the balloons with the following sentences:

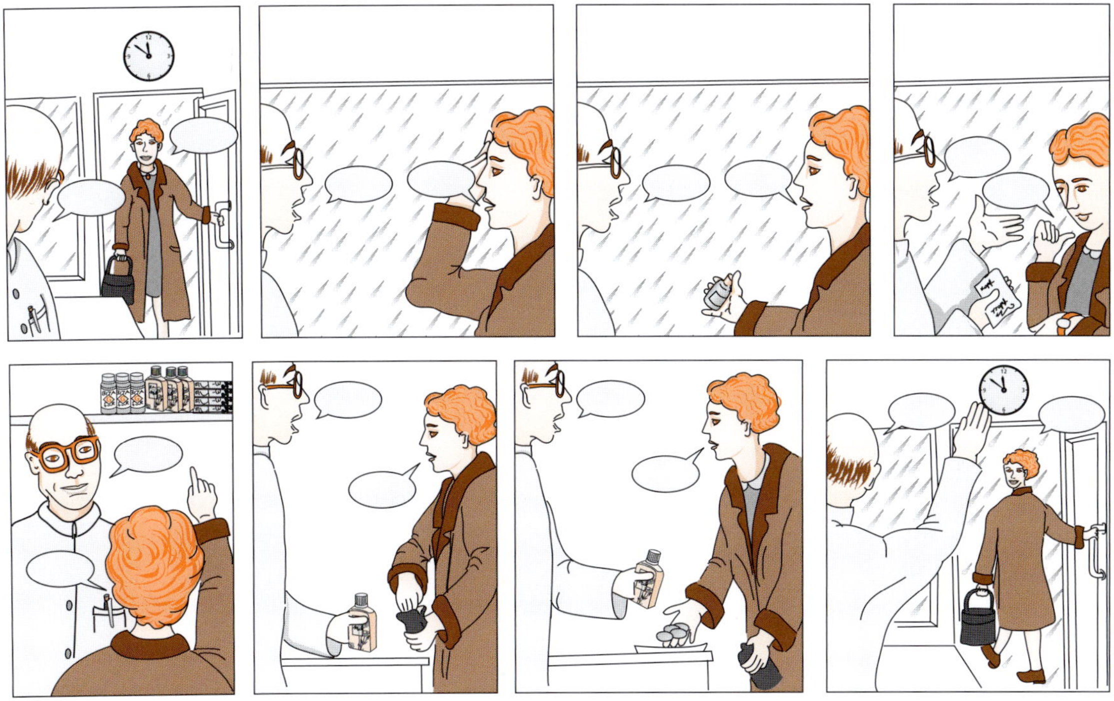

Thank you, bye-bye.

What can I do for you?

Yes, please, I'd like a small bottle of that mild after-shave lotion.

How much is it, please?

Not so well, I'm feeling the weather.

Thank you very much. I wish you a speedy recovery.

I'm sorry, but you need a prescription for that medicine. Anyway, it would be better for you to consult a doctor.

It costs € 8.95, please.

Here you are.

You are right. I'll try to see the doctor this afternoon.

Here you are.

How are you today?

Hello, Mr Johnson.

Good morning, Mrs Bradley.

Could you give me those drops I had last time for my heart trouble?

Is there anything else I can do for you?

2. Complete this dialogue:

Chemist:	**Customer:**
Hello	Good afternoon.
What can I do for you	My doctor gave me this prescription.
Sorry I must order this medicine	Alright, then I'll come back tomorrow. When will your pharmacy be open? Tomorrow is Saturday.
from 8am to 1pm	I see, then I'll come back tomorrow morning.
Can I do something else for you	Yes, please, have you got baby food?
Yes, how old is the baby	5 months.
Which kind of food do you like	I'll take two jars of carrots.
Here you are	Thank you, how much is it?
2,95 $	Here you are. Bye, bye. See you tomorrow.
thank you bye	

3. Can you explain the way?

You are working at the pharmacy in Old Street.

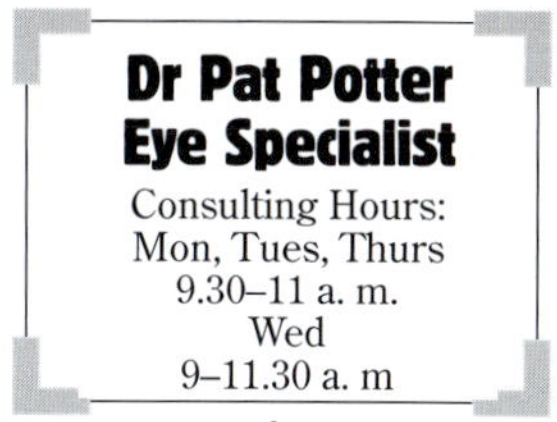

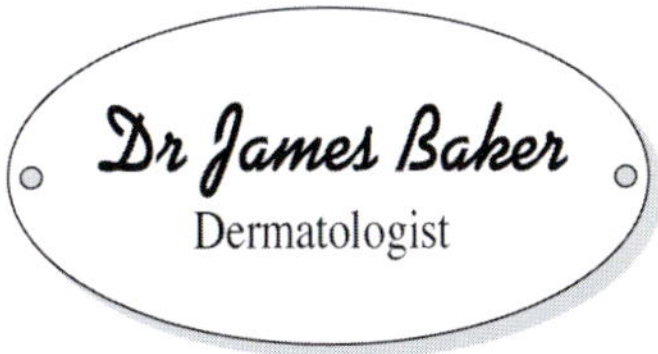

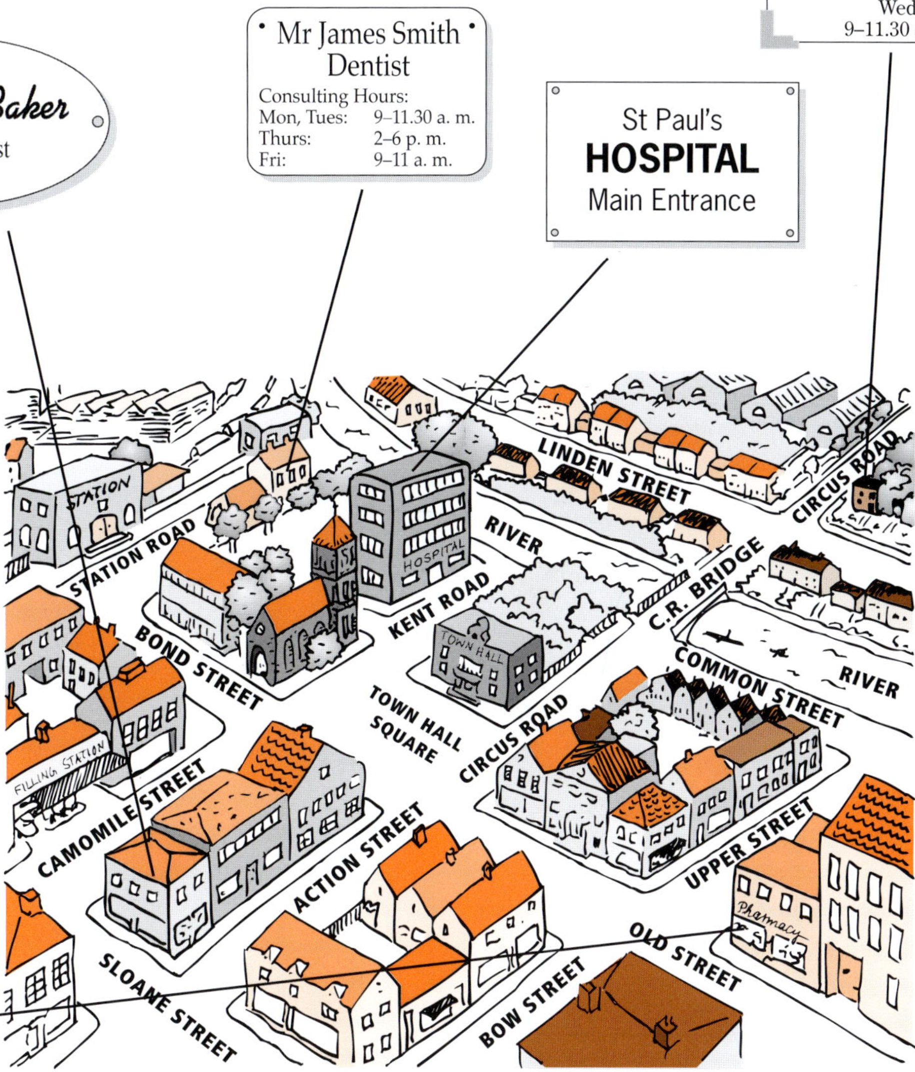

a) Explain to customer A the way to the nearest dentist.
b) Customer B wants to know the way to the dermatologist.
c) Customer C has to go to hospital. Tell him where it is.
d) Customer D asks for an eye specialist. Explain to him the way to Dr Potter's practice.

4. Can you make a dialogue?

Chemist	**Customer**
Mehrere Kunden befinden sich in der Apotheke. Sie fragen, wer an der Reihe ist. Who is next	Es meldet sich die alte Stammkundin Mrs Barker.
Sie begrüßen sie freundlich und fragen, was sie tun können. Hello, what can I do for you?	Mrs Barker überreicht Ihnen ein Rezept für eine Rheumasalbe.
Sie erklären, dass die Salbe erst zubereitet werden müsse, und bitten die Kundin, kurz Platz zu nehmen. The oitment must be prepaired can you take a sit	Die Kundin bedankt sich, zumal sie sich ein wenig schwach auf den Beinen fühle.
Sie empfehlen ihr, dass sie auf sich achtgeben solle, denn sie sähe etwas blass aus. Take care of you you are very pale	Mrs Barker erklärt, dass sie seit heute morgen auch noch Zahnschmerzen hätte.
Sie erzählen, dass sich ein neuer Zahnarzt in der Gegend niedergelassen hätte und erklären den Weg zu seiner Praxis.	Die Kundin sagt, dass sie ihn demnächst mal aufsuchen werde.
Die Salbe ist fertig. Sie überreichen sie Mrs Barker und fragen nach weiteren Wünschen.	Mrs Barker verlangt noch Kohletabletten und Mundwasser.
Sie geben ihr beides.	Die Kundin bedankt sich und fragt, was sie schuldig sei.
Sie nennen den Betrag.	Die Kundin gibt Ihnen das Geld.
Sie geben das Wechselgeld zurück, bedanken sich und wünschen gute Besserung.	

Part two

1. Do you understand these directions?

SURGICAL SPIRIT

For medical purposes only.

CAUTION: This preparation is inflammable, keep away from naked flame. Not to be taken!

LAXEASY

The effortless laxative LAXEASY is a blend of milk of magnesia and an ultrafine grade of medical paraffin for the gentle relief of constipation – exactly what is needed when you must avoid strain or effort. This is why LAXEASY is so widely used in hospitals and nursing homes.

When to use: Use LAXEASY whenever a quick return to normal habits is desired. Because of its gentle action LAXEASY is specially recommended when you are recovering from illness, during pregnancy or if you have piles.

How to use: Shake the bottle well!
Mix dose with half a glass of milk or water if desired.

Adults: 1–2 tablespoonfuls before breakfast or at bedtime.
Children: 1 year to 7 years: 1–2 teaspoonfuls at bedtime.
over 7 years: 1/2–1 tablespoonful at bedtime.
Babies: LAXEASY should be given under medical advice.

MENTHOLATUM Greaseless – stainless – pleasant smelling
Extra strong for faster results

Massage Mentholatum into the affected part until it is absorbed by the skin. Repeat at least every two hours. This extra-strong combination of proven medicaments brings faster relief from rheumatic pain, muscular stiffness and strain, chest-cold discomforts. Leaves no sticky, greasy coating, no stains on clothing or bed linen.

For external use only. – Avoid contact with eyes!

PAINEX-ELIXIR FOR CHILDREN

This medicine should be kept out of reach of children and should not be used to excess.

Dosage: In the absence of specific instructions from your doctor "Painex-Elixir" should be given as follows.
Children: 1 year old or under:
One 5 ml spoonful (preferably in milk).
Children: 2–8 years:
Two 5 ml spoonfuls.
Children over 8 years:
Up to four 5 ml spoonfuls.
The dose may be repeated 4 times a day if required.
Each 5 ml dose contains 120 mg Paracetamol

LIQUID ANTISEPTIC

For all first aid uses and minor ailments, promotes clean, rapid healing. Soothes pain. Fights infections. Reduces swellings.

Keep medicines out of children's reach and out of direct sunlight.

To be used for: Cuts, grazes, bites, stings ...

SUPERPILL
For relief of painful discomfort in the following conditions:

Headaches – Take 1–2 tablets with a glass of water every four hours, as necessary, up to 12 tablets a day.

Colds – Flu – To relieve painful discomfort and reduce fever, take 1 or 2 tablets with a glass of water (or fruit juice) every 4 hours, as necessary, up to 12 tablets a day.

Toothache – Extractions – or for relief of pain following dental treatment, take 1 or 2 tablets with a glass of water every four hours, as necessary, up to 12 tablets a day.

Arthritis and Rheumatism – For the temporary relief of pain, take 1 or 2 tablets with a glass of water every 4 hours, as necessary, up to 12 tablets a day. CAUTION – if pain persists for more than 10 days, or redness is present, or in conditions affecting children unter 12 years of age, consult a physician immediately.

Sore throat due to a cold and for relief of minor throat irritations – To relieve pain and discomfort, take 1 or 2 tablets with a glass of water every four hours, as necessary, up to 12 tablets a day.

Sleeplessness – When caused by minor painful distress or discomfort, take 1 or 2 tablets with a glass of water at bedtime.

NOTE: Your physician may prescribe larger doses, for various conditions, when needed.

WARNING: Keep this and all medicines out of children's reach. In case of accidental overdose, contact a physician immediately.

Universal Liniment

For the relief of rheumatism, lumbago, sciatica, mild sprains, stiffness, tired feet, cramps and chest colds.
Ideal for sportsmen.
Keep out of reach of children
For external use only
Shake the bottle

EXTRA STRONG COUGH MIXTURE

Recommended for coughs, colds, hoarseness and bronchitis.

Dose: Adults, two 5 ml spoonfuls in a little water to be sipped slowly every three or four hours. The recommended dose is to be taken at bedtime.
Shake the bottle

2. Make a dialogue:

Well, I'm not quite sure.

My doctor gave me this prescription. I've had a bad cough since last weekend. It won't go away.

Good morning, sir.

Thank you very much. I hope you feel better and have a nice weekend.

Yes, it's essential to have certain things in the house in case of emergency. Most people forget to replace things in their first aid cupboard. Will that be all?

What can I do for you?

Ah, cough drops. They will help you. Here you are. Quite a few people have been suffering from coughs this winter. Do you know how to take the drops?

That's right. That would be good. Is there anything else I can do for you?

Yes, thank you. How much is it?

Shake the bottle well and take 15 drops on a teaspoonful of sugar or honey every three or four hours.

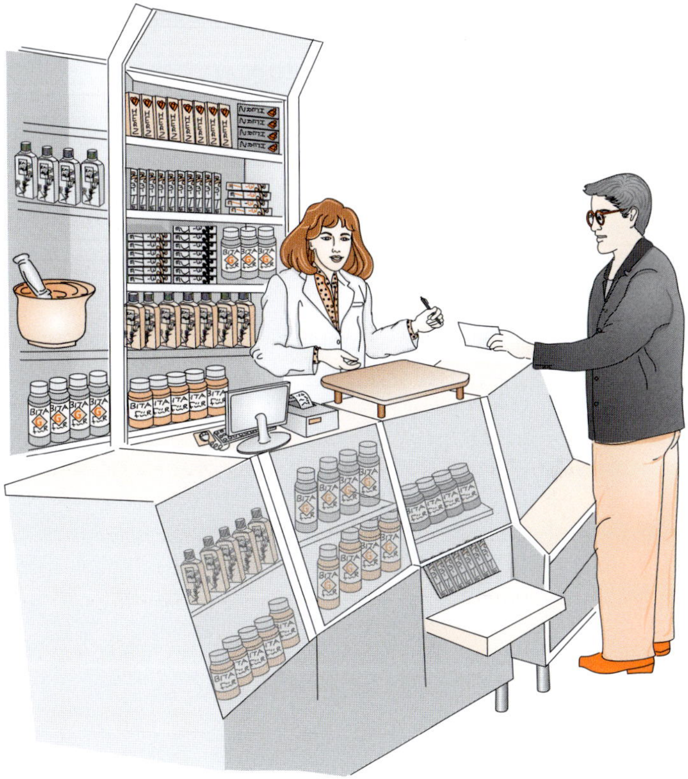

Here you are.

€ 6.80 (six euro eighty), please.

Thanks, goodbye.

Shouldn't I take 15 drops before going to bed?

Good morning, madam.

Some iodine, please, and a strip of plaster, 2.5 cm wide, for my first aid cupboard.

3. Complete this dialogue:

Chemist:	Customer:
	Good morning.
	I hope you can help me. My husband's having trouble with his heart. "Corsan" usually helps him. Have you got some?
	I see, so we've got to see a doctor first. I'll come back this afternoon. When do you close?
	Do you sell diapers?
	Okay, I'll take the small one. How much does it cost?
	Here you are.
	I'll come back this afternoon. Bye-bye.

A few hours later:

Hello.

I’ve got the prescription for “Corsan”.
Here you are.

Yes, he has a travel insurance.

Our daughter’s still a baby.
How much does it cost?

Here you are.

Bye.

4. Can you make a dialogue?

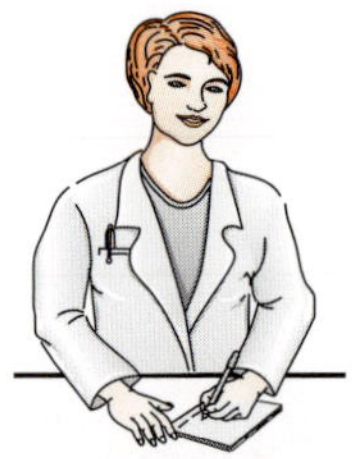

Chemist

Customer

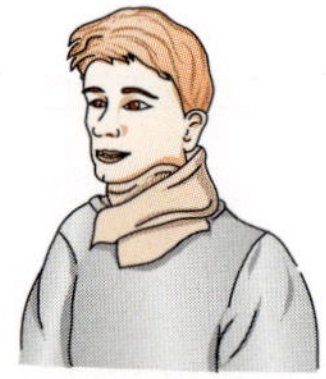

Begrüßen Sie den eintretenden Herrn und fragen Sie, was sie für ihn tun können.

Der Kunde grüßt und sagt, dass er ein Grippemittel und ein schmerzlinderndes Mittel haben wolle.

Sagen Sie, dass viele Leute zur Zeit an Grippe leiden und fragen Sie nach einem Rezept.

Der Kunde gibt dem Apotheker das Rezept und fragt, wie er die beiden Medikamente nehmen soll.

Sagen Sie, dass der Patient von den Grippetabletten 3-mal täglich eine nach den Mahlzeiten nehmen soll und dass die Schmerzmittel Zäpfchen sind, von denen bei auftretenden Schmerzen jeweils eines einzuführen ist. Betonen Sie, dass Medikamente außerhalb der Reichweite von Kindern aufbewahrt werden müssen.

Der Kunde fragt, ob es Schnupfenmittel in Tablettenform gibt.

Sie zeigen eine große und eine kleine Packung und fragen, welche der Herr möchte.

Der Kunde möchte die kleine Packung und fragt, was er schuldig ist.

Sagen Sie wie hoch der Kostenanteil an dem Rezept ist, was die Schnupfentabletten kosten, und fragen Sie, ob Sie sonst noch etwas für ihn tun können.

Der Kunde sagt, dass das alles sei, bezahlt und verabschiedet sich.

Sie wünschen gute Besserung und verabschieden sich ebenfalls.

5. Dialogues:

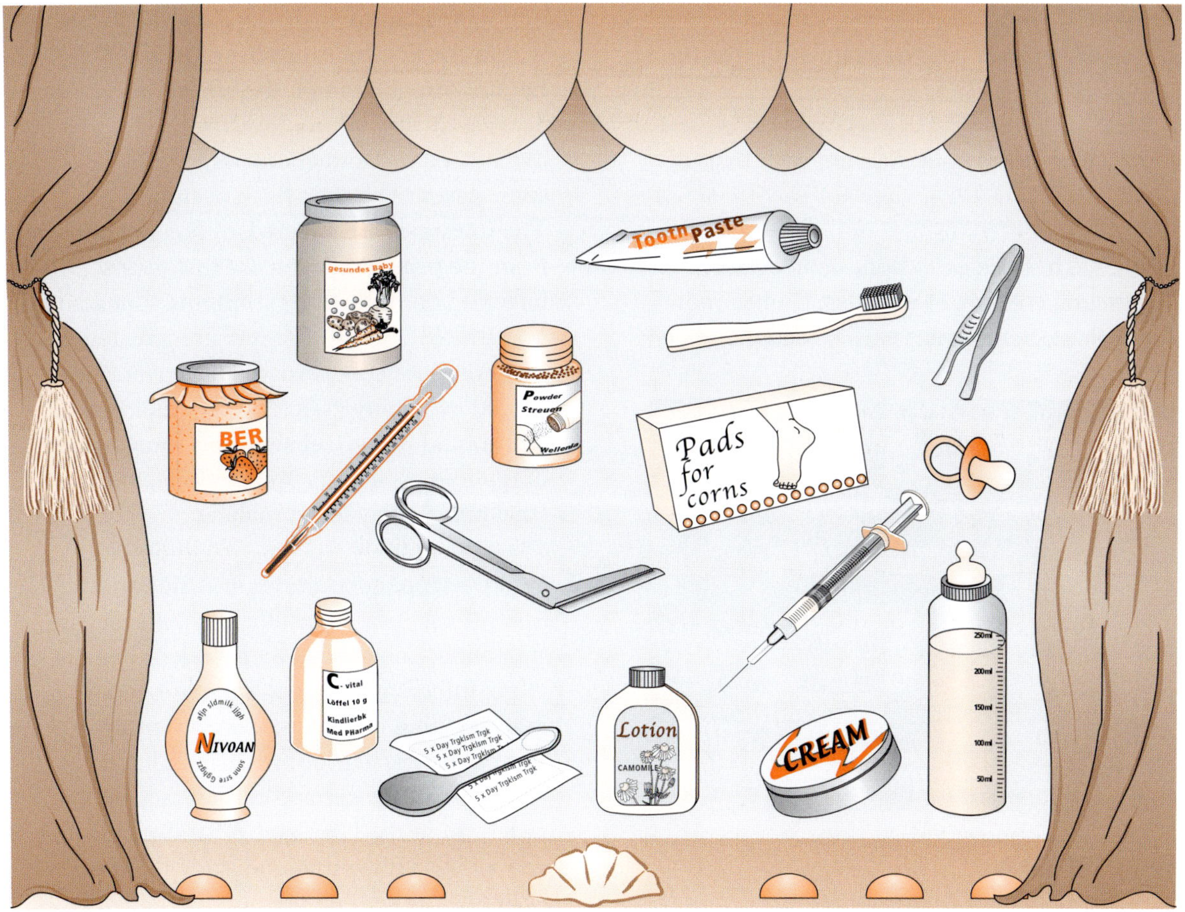

The class is divided up into pairs. Each pair takes a few minutes to put down some notes for a conversation at the chemist's. Practise with your partner. Then one or two pairs perform their dialogues in front of the class.

5.5. Lösungsvorschläge zu den Übungen

Chapter one

1. Please compare your diagram with that on page 3.

2. Please compare your diagram with that on page 5.

3. a) liver, b) freckles, c) bone-marrow, d) spine, vertebral column, e) wrinkles, f) ulna, radius, g) spleen, h) arteries, veins, i) tendon, j) bile

4.

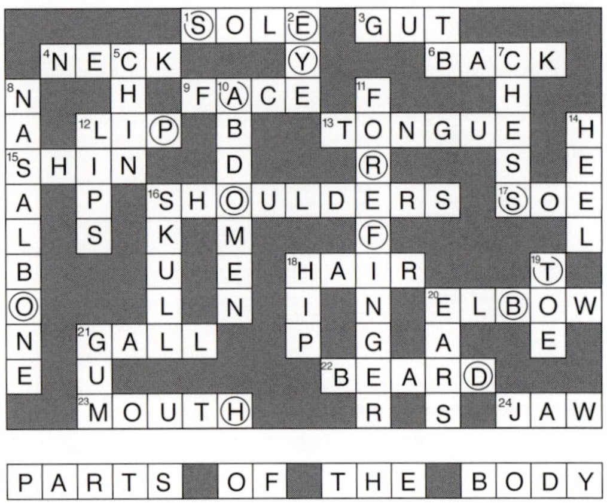

Chapter two

1. a) tonsillitis, b) pneumonia, c) sinusitis, d) bronchitis, e) compare your suggestions with the signs mentioned on page 10.

2. a) 77 °F, 104.5 °F, b) 26.7 °C, 38.2 °C

3. a) measles, German measles, chicken pox, scarlet fever, b) diphtheria, mononucleosis, poliomyelitis, mumps, whooping cough, c) If a pregnant woman catches the disease within the first four months of pregnancy, her unborn child might be affected.

4. a) They come from countries in which some cases of cholera have occurred. b) The intestines are affected. c) It is the period from the time when you are first exposed to infection until the first symptoms appear. d) You should consult a doctor immediately and mention your stay abroad. Furthermore you should avoid any contact with other persons and should be careful about personal hygiene. e) typhoid, dysentery, tuberculosis, meningitis, smallpox, yellow fever, malaria.

5. a) in developing countries in Africa and South-East Asia, b) insufficient medical care, starvation, unbalanced diets, lack of hygiene, c) no. Infectious diseases are more common in developing countries; there are more cancers and cardiovascular disorders in industrialized countries, d) cancer and cardiovascular disorders, e) in the USA and Australia, f) similar way of life, unhealthy food, stressful jobs, pollution, g) high cholesterol level, high blood pressure, smoking, being overweight, h) there was a decrease in the number of cardiac infarctions during World War II, the increase in the number after the War was perhaps due to the improved standard of living which meant

more fatty food, more money spent on cigarettes, less physical exercise etc., i) people often died from other diseases, j) perhaps pollution, k) no, it wasn't, l) war, famine, epidemics.

6.

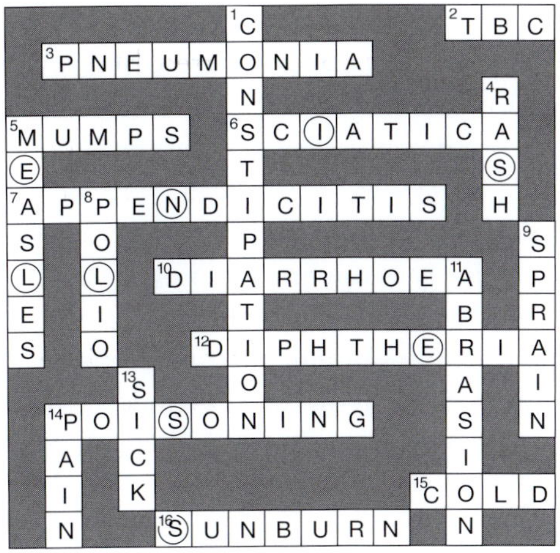

I	L	L	N	E	S	S	E	S

7.

1	A	D	E	N	O	I	D	S	
2	D	I	A	B	E	T	E	S	
3	F	A	I	N	T				
4	C	R	A	M	P				
5	F	R	A	C	T	U	R	E	
6	C	H	O	L	E	R	A		
7	C	O	U	G	H				
8	H	E	A	R	T	B	U	R	N
9	C	A	N	C	E	R			

Chapter three

1. ... some tablets/something to gargle for my sore throat.
   ... painkillers for my toothache.
   ... aspirin for my headache and some suppositories/tablets/cough mixture for my cold.
   ... nose drops.
   ... cough-drops/cough-mixture/sleeping-pills/tablets for insomnia.
   ... some charcoal tablets.
   ... some ointment.

2. 1. teat, 2. dummy, 3. baby powder, 4. tissues, 5. baby cream, 6. bath thermometer, 7. feeding bottle, 8. bottle warmer, 9. baby scales, 10. cotton swabs, 11. nappy, 12. blunt-ended scissors

3. 1b, 2d, 3f, 4a, 5c, 6e

4. TARZAN: a) a series of products, b) before shaving/after shaving, c) to stop body odour.

   DENTY: a) You have to put some drops in a glass, fill it up with water and rinse your mouth and throat. b) It is refreshing and contains essential ingredients. c) They are supposed to reach all parts of the mouth.

   BEAUTY-ADVICE: a) It provides regeneration of the cells, cures irritation of the skin and abrasions. b) vitamins and hormones, c) small quantities are sufficient. d) dust, make-up and impurities, e) You are supposed to add a small quantity to cotton wool and apply it to your face after cleansing. f) Day cream protects the skin against impurities and is an ideal make-up base. Night cream provides constant nourishment for the skin and stimulates the circulation.

5. –
6.

1	S	H	A	M	P	O	O												
2	S	E	D	A	T	I	V	E											
3	L	A	C	T	O	S	E												
4	B	L	U	N	T		E	N	D	E	D								
5	S	T	E	R	I	L	I	Z	I	N	G		T	A	B	L	E	T	S
6	C	H	A	R	C	O	A	L		T	A	B	L	E	T	S			

Chapter four

Part one

1. 1.Good morning, Mrs. Bradley. – Hello, Mr. Johnson. 2. How are you today? – Not so well, I'm feeling the weather. 3. What can I do for you? – Could you give me those drops I had last time for my heart trouble? 4. I'm sorry, but you need a prescription for that medicine. Anyway it would be better to consult a doctor. – You are right. I'll try to see the doctor this afternoon. 5. Is there anything else I can do for you? – Yes please, I'd like a small bottle of that mild after-shave lotion. 6. Here you are. – How much is it, please? 7. It costs € 8.95, please. – Here you are. 8. Thank you very much. I wish you a speedy recovery. – Thank you, bye-bye.

2. Good afternoon. – What can I do for you? – We'll have to order this medicine for you. We'll be open from 9 a.m. till 1 p.m. Can I do anything else for you? – Yes, of course. How old is your baby? – We've got noodles with chicken, beef with peas and tomatoes, carrots ... – Here you are – It costs € 1.75. – Thank you very much. See you tomorrow. Goodbye.

3. 1. Go down Old Street. Cross Town Hall Square. Go along Bond Street and turn right into Station Road. Mr Smith's practice is the first house on the right opposite the station. 2. Go along Old Street. Turn left into Action Street and then right into Sloane Street. Dr Baker's practice is in the first building on the right. 3. Go along Old Street and cross Town Hall Square. Turn right into Kent Road and you'll find the hospital on the left(-hand side). 4. Turn right into Upper Street, then first left into Common Street. At the end turn right and cross the bridge. Go along Circus Road and you'll find Dr Potter's practice on the right(-hand side).

4. Who's next? – I am/Hello, Mrs. Barker. What can I do for you? – Hello. My doctor gave me this prescription for some ointment for my rheumatism/Your ointment will have to be made up. Would you take a seat, please, for a few minutes. – Oh yes, thank you, I'm feeling a little weak in my legs today/You must look after yourself, Mrs Barker. You look very pale. – I've had terrible toothache since this morning/There's a new dentist not far from here. His practice is opposite the station. You

just go down Old Street ... – Fine. I'll try and make an appointment with him in the next few days/Your ointment is ready. Here you are. Can I do anything else for you? – Oh yes, I'd like some charcoal tablets and some mouthwash, please/Here you are. – Thank you very much. How much do I owe you?/€ 7.40 (seven euro fourty), please, Mrs Barker. – Here you are/ Thank you. Your change, Mrs. Barker. I hope you feel better soon. – Thank you, bye-bye.

Part two

1. –
2. Good morning, sir. – Good morning, madam. What can I do for you? – My doctor gave me this prescription. I've had a bad cough since last weekend. It won't go away./Ah, cough drops, they will help you. Here you are. Quite a few people have been suffering from coughs this winter. Do you know how to take the drops? – Well, I'm not quite sure./Shake the bottle well and take 15 drops on a teaspoonful of sugar or honey every three or four hours. – Shouldn't I take 15 drops before going to bed?/That's right. That would be good. Is there anything else I can do for you? – Some iodine, please, and a strip of plaster, 2.5 cm wide, for my first aid cupboard. Yes, it's essential to have certain things in the house in case of emergency. Most people forget to replace things in their first aid cupboard. Will that be all? – Yes, thank you, how much is it?/€ 6.80 (six euro eighty), please. – Here you are./Thank you very much. I hope you feel better and have a nice weekend. – Thanks, goodbye.
3. Good morning. – What can I do for you? – We've got some, but you need a prescription. – We close at 6.30. Is there anything else I can do for you? – Yes, we do. We've got large and small packets. – € 9.50 (nine euro fifty), please. – Thank you very much, goodbye. – Good afternoon. – What can I do for you? – Thank you. Has your husband got a health insurance? – Keep this medicine away from children. – You have to pay € 8.00, please. – Thank you, bye-bye.
4. Good afternoon, sir. What can I do for you? – Good afternoon, could you give me something for flu and some painkillers./ A lot of people have flu at the moment. Have you got a prescription? – Yes, I have. Here you are. How should I take these tablets?/ Take one of these tablets for the flu three times a day after meals. The painkillers are suppositories. Insert one in the rectum, whenever the pain comes on. Please keep them away from children. – Have you got something to stop catarrh?/Large or small. Which would you like? – I'll take the small one. How much do I owe you? / € 3.00 for the prescription and the pills cost 3.90. € 6.90 altogether. Is there anything else I can do for you? – No thank you, that's all. Here you are. – Goodbye. I hope you feel better soon. Goodbye.
5. –

a) can – could – to be able to
b) may – might – to be allowed to

Grammar

6

In diesem Abschnitt sollen einige wichtige Grammatikstrukturen anhand von Beispielen aus dem Bereich der Apotheke wieder ins Gedächtnis gerufen werden. Zu jedem Abschnitt finden Sie Übungen im Übungsteil ab Seite 82.

6.1. Questions

a) Fragen mit Hilfsverben (auxiliary verbs)

Is your husband ill?
Should I stay in bed?
Are you feeling better today?
Can you come later?
When **can** you come?
What **am** I allowed to eat?
Whose turn **is** it?
Have you taken your temperature?

Fragen, die ein Hilfsverb enthalten, benötigen keine Umschreibung mit to do, unabhängig davon, ob es sich um Entscheidungsfragen (*1) oder um Fragewortfragen handelt.

*1) Entscheidungsfragen sind Fragen, die mit 'ja' oder 'nein' beantwortet werden.

b) Fragen mit **to do**-Umschreibung

Do you know how to take these tablets?
Did you take the drops regularly?
Doesn't your sister feel well?
What kind of pills **did** you take?
Which doctor **did** you consult?
When **do** you go back to work?
Do you have a prescription? (*2)

*2) 'have' kann ein Hilfsverb (letztes Beispiel unter a) oder ein Vollverb (letztes Beispiel unter b) sein. 'Have' als Vollverb wird mit to do umschrieben.

Fragen, die kein Hilfsverb enthalten, benötigen die Umschreibung mit to **do**, wiederum unabhängig davon, ob es sich um Entscheidungsfragen oder um Fragewortfragen handelt.

c) Fragen, die nach dem Subjekt oder einem Teil des Subjekts fragen:

Who caught a cold?
What helped you to get rid of your cough?
Which customer brought this prescription?

Ausnahme: Fragesätze, die nach dem Subjekt oder einem Teil des Subjekts fragen, brauchen keine Umschreibung mit to do. Die folgenden Fragewörter können eine solche Subjektfrage einleiten: who – what – which – how many – how much – whose.

6.2. Negative sentences

Auf die Verneinung soll nur kurz eingegangen werden, da hier die gleichen Regeln gelten wie für den Fragesatz:

a) Verneinte Sätze mit Hilfsverb

I **cannot** sleep at night.
I **haven't** had a cold for two years.
Dr Smith **is** not at home.

> Verneinte Sätze, die ein Hilfsverb enthalten benötigen keine Umschreibung mit to do.

b) Verneinte Sätze mit **to do**-Umschreibung

Jim **doesn't** want to stay in bed.
He **didn't** go to school today.
I **don't** take any tablets at all.

> Verneinte Sätze ohne Hilfsverb müssen mit to do umschrieben werden.

6.3. Auxiliaries

a) **can – could – to be able to**

You can get painkillers at the chemist's.	Sie können Schmerzmittel in der Apotheke bekommen.
Dr Walter couldn't come yesterday.	Herr Dr. Walter konnte gestern nicht kommen.
He could come tomorrow.	Er könnte morgen kommen.
He will be able to relieve the pain.	Er wird Ihre Schmerzen lindern können.

> can = können, imstande sein
> could = konnte oder auch könnte
> Andere Zeitformen müssen mit der Ersatzform **to be able to** gebildet werden.

b) **may – might – to be allowed to**

May I help you?	Darf/Kann ich Ihnen helfen?
Dr Walter **may** be able to help you.	Herr Dr. Walter kann Ihnen vielleicht helfen.
Has she **been allowed to** leave the house?	Darf sie das Haus verlassen?
She **might** not be able to swallow these capsules.	Sie kann diese Tabletten vielleicht nicht schlucken.

may = darf, kann (im Sinne von "darf"); eine andere Bedeutung ist "vielleicht";
may not hat fast immer die Bedeutung vielleicht nicht;
"nicht dürfen" wird meistens mit **must not** oder **not to be allowed to** übersetzt;
to be allowed to ist die Ersatzform für **may** im Sinne von dürfen;
might = (könnte) vielleicht;
"durfte" wird immer mit **was allowed to** übersetzt.

c) **shall – to be to – to be said to – should – to be supposed to**

*3) 'to be supposed to' hat die gleiche Bedeutung wie 'to be said to'

Shall I go to the chemist's?	Soll ich zur Apotheke gehen?
I am to make up this ointment for Mrs Brickley.	Ich soll diese Salbe für Mrs Brickley zubereiten.
Dr Smith is said to be (*3) an excellent dentist.	Herr Dr. Smith soll eine ausgezeichneter Zahnarzt sein.
You shouldn't drink so much coffee.	Du solltest nicht so viel Kaffee trinken.
You ought to stay in bed.	Du solltest eigentlich im Bett bleiben.

shall = "soll" wird nur in Fragesätzen in der 1. Person (ich, wir) verwendet.
to be to ist die Ersatzform für "sollen", wenn es sich um eine Anweisung handelt.
to be said to heißt "sollen" im Sinne eines Gerüchts.
should und ought to = "sollte" drückt eine Verpflichtung oder einen Ratschlag aus.

d) **must – must not – to have to**

I **must** go to the dentist.	Ich muss zum Zahnarzt gehen.
You **must not** drink too much beer.	Du darfst nicht zu viel Bier trinken.
I **have to** send this prescription to my insurance company.	Ich muss dieses Rezept zu meiner Versicherung senden.

must = muss;
die Ersatzform lautet **to have to**;
must not heißt immer "darf nicht";
die Ersatzform dafür heißt **not to be allowed to**.

e) **need**

He **needn't** call the doctor. I feel better already.	Er braucht den Arzt nicht zu rufen. Ich fühle mich schon besser.
Need I fill in this form?	Muss ich dieses Formular ausfüllen?
The chemist **needs** the prescription.	Der Apotheker braucht das Rezept.

need kann Hilfsverb und Vollverb sein. Als Hilfsverb kommt es nur in Frage und Verneinung vor. Es braucht keine Umschreibung mit **to do** und kein "s" in der 3. Person Singular.
Ein folgender Infinitiv wird ohne **"to"** angeschlossen.
Als Vollverb kommt **need** auch im bejahten Aussagesatz vor, braucht die **to do**-Umschreibung, das "s" in der 3. Person Singular und kann alle Zeiten bilden.

6.4. Past Tense and Present Perfect

a) Spanish Flu affected over 500 million people between 1918 and 1922.

Past Tense (Imperfekt) wird zur Darstellung von Handlungen verwendet, die in der Vergangenheit abgeschlossen wurden, insbesondere dann, wenn der Satz eine Zeitbestimmung enthält, die keinen Bezug zur Gegenwart hat **(yesterday, in 1945 ...)**

b) There **have been** enormous advances in medicine **since 1945**.
c) I **haven't consulted** a doctor **for over three years**.

Das **Present Perfect** (Perfekt) steht bei Handlungen, die in der Vergangenheit angefangen haben und bis in die Gegenwart fortdauern, bzw. deren Auswirkungen für die Gegenwart von Bedeutung sind. Dies wird besonders deutlich, wenn der Satz Zeitbestimmungen enthält, die den Bezug zur Gegenwart betonen **(since, for (*4), up to now, not yet ...)**

Im Deutschen werden Imperfekt und Perfekt gleichbedeutend verwendet. Statt des englischen Present Perfect steht häufig die Gegenwart. Eine Liste der unregelmäßigen Verben befindet sich im Kap. 7.4.

*4) since = 'seit' steht für 'von einem bestimmten Zeitpunkt an', während for = 'seit' 'während eines bestimmten Zeitraums' bedeutet.

6.5. Conditional clauses

a) **If** you give up smoking, you will feel better.
If you suffer from toothache, you must consult a dentist.

Die beiden Beispiele unter a) stellen Bedingungen dar, die der Sprecher für erfüllbar hält. Der **If**-Satz steht dabei in der **Gegenwart**, der **Hauptsatz** im **Futur**. Anstelle von **will** kann auch ein anderes Hilfsverb stehen.

b) **If** you **gave up** smoking, you **would get rid of** that cough.
If I **knew** Dr Potter's phone number, I **could ring** him.

Der erste Satz unter b) stellt eine aus der Perspektive des Sprechers nur vorgestellte, der zweite Satz eine unerfüllbare Bedingung dar. Der **If**-Satz steht hier im **Past Tense**, der **Hauptsatz** im **conditonal (would + Infinitiv)**. Anstelle von **would** kann auch **could** oder **might** stehen, wenn es der Sinn erlaubt.

c) If she **had stayed** in bed, she **wouldn't have suffered** a relapse.

Beispielsatz c) stellt eine unerfüllbare Bedingung dar, da Bedingung und Folge bereits in der Vergangenheit stattgefunden haben. In diesem Fall steht der **If-Satz** im **Past Perfect** und der **Hauptsatz** im **Conditional Perfect (would have + past participle)**.

6.6. Reported speech

"My wife also **had** problems with her stomach."
"Now she **drinks** a cup of fennel tea every evening and **feels** much better."
"I'm sure fennel tea **will help** you, too."

a) **The chemist says** that his wife also **had** problems with her stomach.
that now she **drinks** a cup of fennel tea every evening and **feels** much better.
that he is sure fennel tea **will help** me, too.

Steht der Hauptsatz in der Gegenwart (*5), so steht im Nebensatz (indirekte Rede) dieselbe Zeit wie in der direkten Rede.

*5) Dieselbe Regel gilt auch, wenn der Hauptsatz im Present Perfect (The chemist has said) oder im Futur (The chemist will tell me) steht.

b) **The chemist said** that his wife **had** also **had** problems with her stomach.
that now she **drank** a cup of fennel tea every evening and **felt** much better.
that he is sure fennel tea **would help** me, too.

Steht der Hauptsatz im Past, so verändern sich die Zeiten im Nebensatz folgendermaßen:

direkte Rede:		**indirekte Rede:**
Präsens	→	Past
Past, Present Perfect	→	Past Perfect
Futur	→	Conditional

6.7. The passive voice

a) **We sell these drops** very often. — **These drops are sold** very often (by us).
The chemist gave the tablets to the customer. — **The tablets were given** to the customer (by the chemist).

Wie im Deutschen können auch im Englischen aktive Sätze, die ein Akkusativobjekt enthalten, in einen Passivsatz umgewandelt werden. Das **Akkusativobjekt** des **Aktivsatze**s wird zum **Subjekt des Passivsatzes**. Das Subjekt des Aktivsatzes kann mit **by** angehängt werden, wird aber häufig weggelassen, wenn es nicht unbedingt erforderlich ist.

b) **We are offering all customers little presents** today. — **Little presents are being offered** to all customers today.
All customers are being offered little presents today.

They looked after grandma while we were on holiday. — **Grandma was looked after** while we were on holiday.

Häufiger als im Deutschen wird im Englischen auch ein **Dativobjekt** zum **Subjekt eines Passivsatze**s gemacht. (*6) Da der erste Aktivsatz in Beispiel b) ein Dativ- und ein Akkusativobjekt enthält, sind also zwei Passivkonstruktionen möglich. Abweichend vom Deutschen kann auch das präpositionale Objekt zum Subjekt eines Passivsatzes werden.

*6) Dieser persönliche Passiv wird im Deutschen häufig mit einer unpersönlichen Konstruktion übersetzt (Man bot allen Kunden ...)

6.8. Relative clauses

Personenbezogene Relativpronomen:

a) The customer **who/that** had forgotten his prescription returned in the afternoon.
b) The dermatologist **whom/who/that** Mr. Miller had recommended was on holiday.
c) The eye specialist **whom/who/that** John asked for was not in his office.
d) Customers **whose** medicines have to be made up can take a seat over there.

*7) Beispielsatz c) könnte auch lauten: The eye specialist for whom John asked ... In diesem Fall muss das Relativpronomen whom verwendet werden.

In der Schriftsprache lautet das personenbezogene Relativpronomen im 1. Fall (Beispiel a) **who**, im 4. Fall (Beispiel b) **whom**, bei Präpositionen (Beispiel c) ebenfalls **whom** (*7). In der Umgangssprache wird in den Beispielsätzen b) und c) **who** oder das Weglassen des Relativpronomens bevorzugt. Für **whose** gibt es keine Varianten.

Sachbezogene Relativpronomen:

a) Mumps is a disease **which/that** can be quite serious for adults.
b) The medicine **which/that/** – we ordered for you hasn't come yet.
c) Cancer is a disease **which/that/** – nobody likes to think about. (*8)
d) Remedies **whose** side effects have not been tested carefully should not be sold.
Remedies the side effects **of which** have not been tested carefully should not be sold.

*8) Auch hier könnte man den Satz umstellen: Cancer is a disease about which nobody likes to think.

Die Schriftsprache verwendet in den Beispielsätzen a), b) und c) **which** als sachbezogenes Personalpronomen. In der Umgangssprache bevorzugt man **that** oder lässt das Pronomen weg. **Whose** (Beispielsatz d) kann auch bei Sachen stehen. Etwas altmodisch ist die Konstruktion mit **of which**.

A sun lotion, **which you can find on the shelf over there**, will protect your skin.
Dr Smith, **whose office is next door**, came in this morning.

Bei Relativsätzen, deren Inhalt nur eine erläuternde, für den Hauptsatz nicht unbedingt notwendige Aussage erhält, darf das Relativpronomen nicht weggelassen werden. Ferner müssen sie durch Kommas vom Hauptsatz abgetrennt werden. (*9)

*9) Diese Art von Relativsätzen sind weitaus seltener als die bisher beschriebenen notwendigen Relativsätze.

6.9. Adjectives and adverbs

a) Stephen had a **terrible** pain.
The pain was **terrible**.

b) The driver of the blue Ford didn't drive **carefully**.
Stephen was not **particularly** careful either.
In fact, the blue Ford drove along **extremely** quickly.
Stephen **usually** left home ten minutes earlier.

Adjektive treten auf als
- Ergänzungen zu einem Substantiv wie im ersten Beispiel oder
- mit einer Form von to be als Teil des Prädikats wie im zweiten Beispiel unter a)

Adverbien treten auf als
- nähere Bestimmung eines Verbs (1. Satz unter b)
- nähere Bestimmung eines Adjektivs (2. Satz unter b)
- nähere Bestimmung eines anderen Adverbs (3. Satz unter b)
- nähere Bestimmung eines ganzen Satzes (4. Satz unter b)

Einige Adjektive können unverändert als Adverb übernommen werden: **fast, long, straight, early, hourly, daily, weekly, hard** (*10)
z. B.: Don't forget to take your tablets **daily**.

*10) hardly heißt kaum

Nach einigen Verben steht ein Adjektiv anstelle eines Adverbs:
to feel (awful), to look (pale), to taste (good), to smell (bad), to get (dark), to become (rich), to stay (poor), to sound (strange)

6.10. Grammar exercises

1. Questions

Fragen Sie nach den fett gedruckten Sätzen bzw. Satzteilen:

a) She is allowed to eat **everything**.
b) **Dr Smith** came in the afternoon.
c) **He takes the tablets regularly.**
d) Your mother should buy **a new dummy**.
e) **Dr Morton is an excellent paediatrician.**
f) Mrs. Jenkins is **my** best customer.
g) We took **Stephen** to the X-ray department.
h) He recommended the **smaller** package.
i) Your husband must take **three** tablets a day.

2. Negative Sentences

Verneinen Sie folgende Sätze:

a) I can sleep during the day.
b) He felt alright this morning.
c) My father wants to stay in bed.
d) I've had a cough for almost three months.
e) The pharmacy will be closed this afternoon.
f) The chemist recommended charcoal tablets.

3. Auxiliaries

Setzen Sie ein passendes Verb bzw. Hilfszeitwort ein:

a) Du musst zum Arzt gehen.
You ______ go to the doctor.
b) Vielleicht leidet das Baby an Blähungen.
The baby ______ suffer from wind.
c) Darf ich aufstehen?
______ I get up?
d) Könnten Sie bitte einen Arzt rufen.
______ you call a doctor, please.
e) Man braucht für dieses Medikament kein Rezept.
You ______ a prescription for this remedy.
f) Mein Mann durfte keinen Kaffee trinken.
My husband ______ to drink coffee.
g) Er würde nicht zur Apotheke gehen können.
He ______ to go to the chemist's.
h) Ich musste morgens eine Tablette nehmen.
I ______ take one tablet in the morning.
i) Du solltest das Rauchen eigentlich aufgeben.
You ______ give up smoking.

4. Past Tense and Present Perfect

Setzen Sie das Verb in Klammern in die richtige Zeit:

a) I (to have) this cough since we came back from Spain.
b) Jane (to have) terrible flu, when we were in Italy.
c) Dr Wesker (to be running) this chemist's shop for over three years now.
d) In London we immediately (to look for) a chemist's shop.
e) Julian (to be) taken to hospital this morning.
f) I (to be waiting) for this remedy for over 10 minutes now.

5. Conditional clauses

Setzen Sie die Verben in die richtige Form.

a) If you (to take) these tablets regularly, your cough will disappear within a few days.
b) You wouldn't have to stay in bed, if you (to have) no fever.
c) Peter (to feel) better, if his diet was healthier.
d) He would have taken these drops, if his doctor (to prescribe) them.
e) If our pharmacy was open during the whole day, Mr Smith (to be able to come) at 2 p.m.
f) This tooth won't hurt any longer, if you (to go) to the dentist.

6. Reported speech

Bilden Sie eine indirekte aus der folgenden direkten Rede.

Tony said: "I will get these remedies from the chemist's. His shop is open the whole day. He was on holiday, but he came back last Friday".

Tony said that

7. The passive voice

Setzen Sie im folgenden die Passivsätze in das Aktiv und die Aktivsätze in das Passiv. Bilden Sie zwei Passivsätze, wenn es möglich ist.

a) This ointment must be made up by a chemist.
b) Yesterday Dr Marlowe gave her the prescription.
c) They will charge me € 3.50 for the tablets.
d) She asked the customer, whether he knew how to take the tablets.
e) He had been told by his doctor that he should stay in bed.
f) Did I tell you that they now close the shop from 1 p.m. to 3 p.m.?

8. Relative clauses

Vervollständigen Sie die folgenden Sätze durch Relativpronomen. Wo kann das Relativpronomen entfallen?

a) The pills ______ your doctor recommended are no longer available.
b) I know someone ______ takes these drops regularly.
c) The chemist ______ shop is round the corner had a bad accident.
d) At the beginning of this century there was a flu epidemic ______ killed thousands of people.
e) Whooping cough is a serious cough (from) ______ mainly children suffer (from).
f) This is the man (to) ______ I gave the drops (to).
g) There are countries in ______ remedies are sold (______) side-effects have not been tested.
h) The dentist ______ I consulted twice a year has retired.

9. Adjectives and adverbs

Entscheiden Sie, ob in den folgenden Sätzen ein Adjektiv oder ein Adverb stehen muss. Bilden Sie gegebenenfalls die richtige Adverbform.

a) Your (daily) dose should not exceed 5 tablets.
b) Your mother looked rather (pale), when I saw her this morning.
c) Please open the ampule (careful).
d) Dr Webster is a very (careful) physician.
e) I won't consult Dr Roger again. Last time I had to wait (extreme) (long).

6.11. Lösungsvorschläge zu den Grammatikübungen

1. a) What is she allowed to eat?
   b) Who came in the afternoon?
   c) Does he take the tablets regularly?
   d) What should your mother buy?
   e) Is Dr Morton an excellent paediatrician?
   f) Whose best customer is Mrs Jenkins?
   g) Whom did we take to the X-ray department?
   h) Which package did he recommend?
   i) How many tablets does your husband have to take/must your husband take?

2. a) I can't sleep ...
   b) He didn't feel alright ...
   c) My father doesn't want to stay ...
   d) I haven't had a cough ...
   e) The pharmacy won't be closed ...
   f) The chemist didn't recommend ...

3. a) must/have to b) might c) May d) Could e) don't need f) was not allowed g) would not be able h) had to i) ought to

4. a) have had b) had c) has been running d) looked for e) was f) have been waiting

5. a) take b) had c) would feel d) had prescribed e) would be able to come f) go

6. ... he would get. ... was open ... He had been ... he had come back the Friday before.

7. a) A chemist must be made up this ointment.
   b) Yesterday she was given the prescription by Dr M./Yesterday the prescription was given to her by Dr M.
   c) I will be charged € 3.50 for the tablets.
   d) The customer was asked whether he knew how to take the tablets.
   e) His doctor had told him that he should stay in bed.
   f) Did I tell you that the shop is now closed from 1 p.m. to 3 p.m.?

8. a) which/that/ –
   b) who
   c) whose
   d) which/that
   e) – /which ... from/from which ...
   f) who(m) ... to/to whom ...
   g) which, whose ...
   h) who(m)/that/ –

9. a) daily b) pale c) carefully d) careful e) an extremely long time

Lösungen

Vocabulary | Wörterverzeichnis

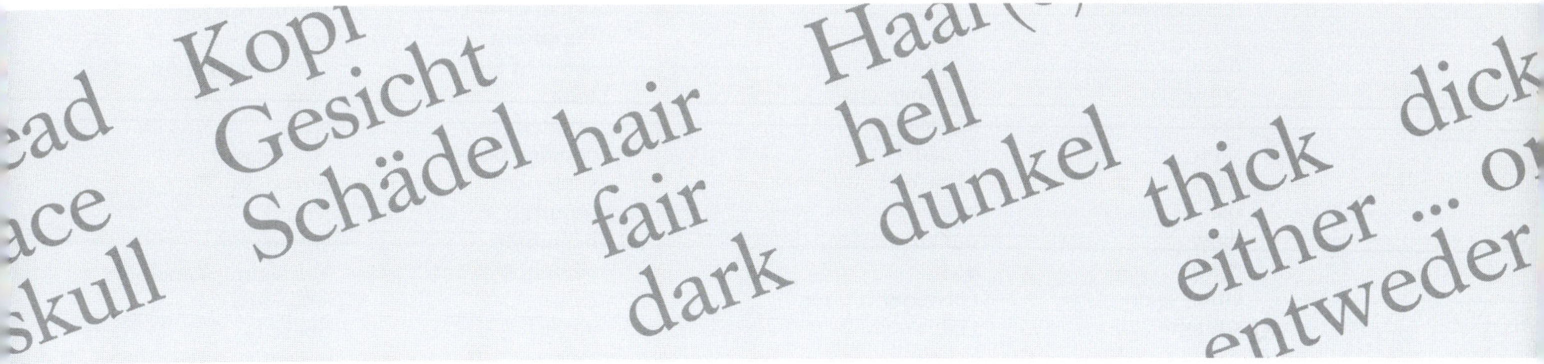

7

7.1. Vocabulary chapter one

The head

head	Kopf
consist of	bestehen aus
face	Gesicht
skull	Schädel
hair	Haar(e)
fair	hell
dark	dunkel
thick	dick
either ... or	entweder ... oder
straight	glatt
parting	Scheitel
curly	lockig
thin	dünn
bald	glatzköpfig
inside	in(nerhalb)
brain	Gehirn
coordinating centre	Koordinationszentrum
nervous system	Nervensystem
side	Seite
control	kontrollieren
opposite	gegenüberliegend
body	Körper
beneath	unter
hair-line	Haaransatz
between	zwischen
temple	Schläfe
forehead	Stirn
see – saw – seen	sehen
eye	Auge
eyelid	Augenlid
eyelashes	Wimpern
eyebrow	Augenbraue
protect	schützen
short-sighted	kurzsichtig
long-sighted, far-sighted	weitsichtig
glasses	Brille
blind	blind
nose	Nase
nostril	Nasenloch
organ of smell	Geruchsorgan
important	wichtig
sense of taste	Geschmackssinn
long	lang
pointed	spitz
aquiline nose	Adlernase
snub nose	Stupsnase
mouth	Mund
beginning	Anfang
alimentary canal	Verdauungskanal
close	schließen
upper	obere(r)
lower	untere(r)
lip	Lippe
tooth – teeth	Zahn – Zähne
jaw	Kiefer
cover	bedecken
gum	Zahnfleisch
tongue	Zunge
food	Essen
organ	Organ
palate	Gaumen
taste buds	Geschmacksknospen
to swallow	schlucken
ear	Ohr
hear – heard – heard	hören
eardrum	Trommelfell
damage	beschädigen
deaf	taub
speak – spoke – spoken	sprechen
mute	stumm
deaf and dumb	taubstumm
communicate	hier: sich verständigen
sign	Zeichen
inner ear	Innenohr
organ of balance	Gleichgewichtsorgan
below	unter

chin	Kinn
grow – grew – grown	wachsen, sich wachsen lassen
beard	Bart
moustache	Schnurrbart
however	jedoch
prefer	bevorzugen
cleanshaven	glattrasiert
uvula	Gaumenzäpfen
cheek	Wange
eye-socket	Augenhöhle
corner of the eye	Augenwinkel
eyeball	Augapfel
iris	Iris
pupil	Pupille

The trunk

neck	Hals
connect	verbinden
trunk	Rumpf
windpipe	Luftröhre
gullet	Speiseröhre
lungs	Lunge
stomach, tummy	Magen
consist of	bestehen aus
shoulder	Schulter
chest	Brustkorb
back	Rücken
buttocks (Pl.)	Gesäß
abdomen, belly	Bauch
whereas	wohingegen
breast	Brust
flat	flach
secrete	absondern
milk	Milch
childbirth	Geburt
slim	schlank
waist	Taille
hip	Hüfte
middle	Mitte
navel	Nabel

The limbs

limbs	Gliedmaßen
arm	Arm
leg	Bein
upper arm	Oberarm
elbow	Ellbogen
forearm	Unterarm
wrist	Handgelenk
hand	Hand
thumb	Daumen
finger	Finger
fingernail	Fingernagel
forefinger, index finger	Zeigefinger
middle finger	Mittelfinger
ring finger, third finger	Ringfinger
little finger	kleiner Finger
remarkable	bemerkenswert
flexibility	Beweglichkeit
enable	befähigen
grasp	greifen
object	Gegenstand
thigh	Oberschenkel
knee	Knie
shin	Schienbein (Körperteil)
calf – calves	Wade
ankle	Knöchel
sprain	verstauchen
foot – feet	Fuß
heel	Ferse
sole	Sohle
toe	Zehe
flat feet	Plattfüße
supports	hier: Einlagen

The skin

skin	Haut
tissue	Gewebe
covering	hier: Umhüllung

smooth	glatt, sanft, weich
puberty	Pubertät
pimple	Pickel
the ... the	je ... desto
put up with	sich abfinden mit
wrinkle	Falte
birthmark	Muttermal
mark	Mal, Zeichen
birth	Geburt
wart	Warze
outgrowth	Auswuchs
develop	entwickeln
viral infection	Virus-Infektion
red-haired	rothaarig
in particular	besonders
freckles	Sommersprossen
cheek	Wange
health	Gesundheit
complexion	Gesichtsfarbe
rosy	rosig
ill, sick	krank
pale	blass

The skeleton

skeleton	Skelett, Knochengerüst
structure	Struktur
internal organ	Inneres Organ
spine, backbone, vertebral column	Wirbelsäule
vertebra	Wirbel
central	zentral
human	menschlich
bone	Knochen
shoulder-blade	Schulterblatt
rib	Rippe
breastbone	Brustbein
radius	Speiche
ulna	Elle
hip-bone	Hüftknochen
knee-cap	Kniescheibe
fibula	Wadenbein
shin-bone, tibia	Schienbein (Knochen)
bone-marrow	Knochenmark
connect	verbinden
joint	Gelenk
sinew, tendon	Sehne
attach	befestigen
muscle	Muskel
confuse	verwechseln
ligament	Band

Some internal organs

heart	Herz
pump	Pumpe
blood	Blut
blood vessel	Blutgefäß
carry	tragen
artery	Arterie
vein	Vene
travel	reisen, hier: fließen
purify	reinigen
liver	Leber
kidney	Niere
gland	Drüse
bile	Galle
gall bladder	Gallenblase
digest	verdauen
fat	fett
absorb	absorbieren
vitamin	Vitamin
task	Aufgabe
regulation	Regulierung
sugar content	Zuckerspiegel
influence	Einfluss
hormone	Hormon
insulin	Insulin
pancreas	Bauchspeicheldrüse
bean-shaped	bohnenförmig
regulate	regulieren
salt	Salz
fluid	Flüssigkeit
level	Niveau, -spiegel

pure	rein
spleen	Milz
be situated	sich befinden
digestive tract	Verdauungstrakt
anus	After
intestine(s), bowel(s), gut	Darm
small intestine	Dünndarm
large intestine	Dickdarm
bladder	(Harn-)Blase

Chapter two

Coughs and colds

cough	Husten, husten (Subst., Verb)
sneeze	Niesen, niesen (Subst., Verb)
common	hier: einfach
cold	Erkältung
general term	allgemeiner Begriff
frequent	häufig
minor	hier: harmlos
illness, sickness, disease	Krankheit
due to	zurückzuführen auf
infection	Infektion
virus	Virus
dangerous	gefährlich
forerunner	Vorläufer
serious	ernst
describe	beschreiben
below	unten
consider to be	betrachten als
flu (influenza)	Grippe
strictly speaking	genau genommen
epidemic	epidemisch, Epidemie
affect	befallen, betreffen, angreifen
die	sterben
sign	Zeichen
ache, pain	Schmerz
headache	Kopfschmerzen
toothache	Zahnschmerzen
stomachache	Bauchschmerzen
hoarseness	Heiserkeit
weariness	Müdigkeit, Mattigkeit
catarrh	Schnupfen
in the case of	im Falle von
fever	Fieber
shivering fit	Schüttelfrost
side effect	Nebenwirkung
sinusitis	Stirnhöhlenkatarrh
inflammation	Entzündung
sinuses	Stirnhöhlen
hollow cavity	Hohlraum
nasal cavity	Nasenhöhle
bone	Knochen
skull	Schädel
accompany	begleiten
tonsillitis	Mandelentzündung
tonsils	Mandeln
swell – swelled – swollen	schwellen
surface	Oberfläche
bronchitis	Bronchitis
bronchial tubes, bronchi	Bronchien
usually	gewöhnlich
cough mixture	Hustensaft
severe	hart, ernst, schwer
lead to – led – led	führen zu
pneumonia	Lungenentzündung
various	verschiedene
type	Art
require	verlangen
careful	vorsichtig, gewissenhaft
nursing	Pflege
appendicitis	Blinddarmentzündung
poliomyelitis	Kinderlähmung
nephritis	Nierenentzündung

Temperature

Monday	Montag
Tuesday	Dienstag
Wednesday	Mittwoch
Thursday	Donnerstag
Friday	Freitag
Saturday	Samstag
Sunday	Sonntag
form	Form
animal	Tier
be unable	nicht in der Lage sein
regulate	regulieren
body temperature	Körpertemperatur
remain	bleiben
hot	heiß
cold	kalt
according to	gemäß
temperature	Temperatur
surroundings	Umgebung
higher	höher
steady	beständig
attack	angreifen
germ	Keim, Bazillus
defence system	Abwehrsystem
increase	wachsen, hier: erhöhen
vary	variieren
raise	heben, hier: erhöhen
excitement	Aufregung
incessant	unaufhörlich
cry	schreien, weinen
class	einstufen
thermometer	Thermometer
reading	(Thermometer)stand
... degrees centigrade	... Grad Celsius

The sick child

sick	krank
child, children	Kind, Kinder
common	hier: üblich
although	obwohl
ignore	außer Acht lassen
disturb	stören
symptom	Symptom
ailment	Gebrechen, Leiden
sweat	schwitzen
shiver	zittern
run a high temperature	eine hohe Temperatur haben
tired	müde
flushed	gerötet
apathetic	apathisch
appetite	Appetit
rash, eruption	Ausschlag
spot	Fleck
appear	erscheinen
scarlet fever	Scharlach
measles	Masern
German measles	Röteln
diarrhoea	Durchfall
indigestion	Verdauungsstörung
constipation	Verstopfung
vomit	erbrechen
result from	herrühren von
variety	Vielzahl
cause	Ursache
sore	wund
throat	Hals, Rachen
diphtheria	Diphtherie
mononucleosis	Pfeiffersches Drüsenfieber
polio(myelitis)	Kinderlähmung
ache	schmerzen
mumps	Mumps
chickenpox	Windpocken
vanish	verschwinden
develop	(sich) entwickeln
spread – spread – spread	(sich) ausbreiten
merge	ineinander übergehen
appearance	Erscheinung

blister	Blase
damp	feucht
armpit	Achsel
groin	Leiste

Vaccination

vaccination	Impfung
protect	schützen
death	Tod
disability	Behinderung
paediatrician	Kinderarzt
recommend	empfehlen
tuberculosis (TB)	Tuberkulose
tetanus	Wundstarrkrampf
whooping cough	Keuchhusten
neurologist	Neurologe
oculist	Augenarzt
orthopaedist	Orthopäde
surgeon	Chirurg
dermatologist	Hautarzt
gynaecologist	Frauenarzt
psychiatrist	Psychiater
general practitioner	Allgemeinmediziner
booster	hier: Auffrischung

Cardiovascular disorders

cardiovascular	Herz- und Gefäß-
disorder	Störung
society	Gesellschaft
developing country	Entwicklungsland
heart attack	Herzattacke
cardiac infarction	Herzinfarkt
death of tissue	Absterben von Gewebe
blood supply	Blutzufuhr
risk factor	Risikofaktor
associate	verbinden
heart trouble	Herzbeschwerden
cholesterol level	Cholesterinspiegel
blood pressure	Blutdruck
overweight	übergewichtig
cigarette smoking	Zigarettenrauchen
increase	erhöhen
risk	Risiko
age	Alter
cause	verursachen
reduce	beeinträchtigen
thrombosis (thromboses)	Thrombose(n)
embolism	Embolie
stroke, apoplectic fit	Schlaganfall
vary	variieren
severity	Ernsthaftigkeit
unconsciousness	Bewusstlosigkeit
paralysis	Lähmung
circulatory	Kreislauf-
constriction of the heart	Herzbeklemmung
occur	auftreten
angina pectoris	Angina pectoris
heart failure	Herzversagen
congenital	angeboren
require	erfordern
operation	Operation
varicose veins	Krampfadern
pregnant	schwanger
irregularity	Unregelmäßigkeit
heartbeat	Herzschlag
nosebleed	Nasenbluten
blow	Schlag
heartburn	Sodbrennen
cirrhosis of the liver	Leberzirrhose
diabetes	Diabetes

Cancers

cancer	Krebs
century	Jahrhundert
inhabitant	Einwohner
life expectancy	Lebenserwartung
die of	sterben an
tumour	Tumor, Geschwulst

malignant	bösartig (Tumor)
site	Stelle
benign	gutartig (Tumor)

Tropical diseases

tropical	tropisch
(be on the) increase	ansteigen
amount	Menge
travel	reisen
the tropics	die Tropen
carelessness	Sorglosigkeit, Unachtsamkeit
precaution	Vorsichtsmaßnahme
cholera	Cholera
case of cholera	Cholerafall
therefore	deshalb
to take precautions	Vorsichtsmaßnahmen ergreifen
interest	Interesse
incubation period	Inkubationszeit
exposure	Ausgesetztsein
appearance	Auftreten
diarrhoea	Durchfall
arrival	Ankunft
recent	kürzlich
stay abroad	Auslandsaufenthalt
avoid	vermeiden
hygiene	Hygiene
spread	Verbreitung
typhoid (fever)	Typhus
typhus	Fleckfieber
dysentery	Ruhr
tuberculosis	Tuberkulose
meningitis	Hirnhautentzündung
smallpox	Pocken
yellow fever	Gelbfieber
malaria	Malaria
affluent	wohlhabend

Additional illnesses

advice	Rat
topic	Thema
holidays	Ferien
South	(in den) Süden
prepare	vorbereiten
remedy	Heilmittel
travel-sickness	Reiseübelkeit
sea-sickness	Seekrankheit
be prone to s.th	zu etwas neigen
to suffer from	leiden an
significant	entscheidend
damage	Schaden
rule	Regel
particularly	besonders
reddening	Erröten
blistering	Blasenbildung
sunburn	Sonnenbrand
sunstroke	Sonnenstich
adequate	angemessen
cover	Bedeckung
cardiac insufficiency	Herzinsuffizienz
heatstroke	Hitzschlag
immediately	sofort
health problem	Gesundheitsproblem
hesitate	zögern
consult	hier: um Rat fragen
sleeplessness	Schlaflosigkeit
goose pimples	Gänsehaut
difficulty in breathing	Atemnot
adenoids	Polypen
collection	(An-)Sammlung
lymphoid tissue	Lymphgewebe
obstruct	behindern
in particula	besonders
suspect	den Verdacht haben
allergy	Allergie
pollen	Pollen
examine	untersuchen
allergic	allergisch

fear	Angst
occasionally	gelegentlich
abdominal pains	Bauchschmerzen
not to agree with	hier: nicht vertragen
explanation	Erklärung
description	Beschreibung
period pains	Menstruationsbeschwerden
agonizing	qualvoll
rule out	ausschließen
gall stones	Gallensteine
painful	schmerzhaft
rheumatism	Rheumatismus
lorrydriver	LKW-Fahrer
carry	tragen
lumbago	Hexenschuss
sciatica	Ischias
backache	Rückenschmerzen
complaint	Beschwerde
medical	medizinisch
rule	Regel
look after	aufpassen auf
lift	heben
bend – bent – bent	beugen
straight	gerade
orthopaedist	Orthopäde
leaflet	Broschüre, Merkblatt
hint	Tipp
suggest	vorschlagen
exercise	Übung
relax	entspannen
pregnancy	Schwangerschaft
piles, haemorrhoids	Hämorrhoiden
remove	entfernen
hospital	Krankenhaus
disappear	verschwinden
prescribe	verschreiben
ointment	Salbe
relief	Erleichterung

Injuries

injury	Verletzung
late	spät
stitches in the side	Seitenstechen
cross	überqueren
regain	wiedergewinnen
consciousness	Bewusstsein
find – found – found	finden
X-ray department	Röntgenabteilung
break – broke – broken	brechen
nurse	Krankenschwester
to be afraid	fürchten
tear – tore – torn	reißen
strain	zerren
guess	raten, hier: ich glaube
operate on s. th.	etw. operieren
prevent	verhindern
stiffness	Steifheit
bruise	blauer Fleck, Quetschung
skin abrasion	Hautabschürfung
moan	stöhnen
concussion	Gehirnerschütterung
explain	erklären
worry	sich Sorgen machen
to fill in a form	ein Formular ausfüllen
admission card	hier: Aufnahmeformular
surname	Nachname
first name	Vorname
marital status	Familienstand
married	verheiratet
single	ledig
widowed	verwitwet
divorced	geschieden
occupation	Beschäftigung, Beruf
next of kin	nächster Verwandter
G. P., general practitioner	praktischer Arzt
venereal disease	Geschlechtskrankheit

migraine	Migräne
bladder	Blase
diabetes	Diabetes
epilepsy	Epilepsie
hepatitis	Hepatitis, Gelbsucht
psychiatric	psychiatrische
treatment	Behandlung
operation	Operation
medication	Verordnung, Medikamente
smoke	rauchen
mental	geistig, seelisch
wheelchair	Rollstuhl
patient	Patient
fall asleep – fell – fallen	einschlafen
burn	Brandwunde
torment	quälen
cramp	Krampf
inflammation of the tendon	Sehnen(scheiden)-entzündung
outpatient	ambulante(r) Patient(in)
rupture of a muscle fibre	Muskelfaserriss
ladder	Leiter
dislocate	ver-, ausrenken
sting – stung – stung	stechen
bite – bit – bitten	beißen

Chapter three

Some common remedies

catch a cold	eine Erkältung bekommen
advice	Ratschlag
a remedy/ medicine for	ein Medikament gegen
reduce	senken, reduzieren
cough drops	Hustentropfen
healthy	gesund
wholemeal bread	Vollkornbrot
vegetable	Gemüse
salad	Salat
laxative	Abführmittel
charcoal tablet	Kohletablette
gargle	Gurgelmittel, gurgeln
prophylactic	vorbeugend, Prophylaktikum
medicine, medicament	Medikament
get addicted to drugs	abhängig werden von Arzneimittel, Rauschgift
pain-killer	Schmerzmittel
tranquillizer, sedative	Beruhigungsmittel
sleeping pill, tablet for insomnia	Schlaftablette
available	erhältlich
prescription	Rezept
customer	Kunde
limited	beschränkt
pharmacology	Pharmakologie
pill	Tablette, Pille
tablet	Tablette, Pille
capsule	Kapsel
granules	Granulat
powder	Pulver, Puder
drops	Tropfen
suppository	Zäpfchen
mixture	Mixtur
cough mixture	Hustensaft
solution	Lösung
emulsion	Emulsion
tincture	Tinktur
ointment	Salbe
cream	Creme
gel	Gel
tea	Tee
ampule	Ampulle
detail	Einzelheit
pharmacopoeia	Arzneibuch

Baby care

baby care	Säuglingspflege
pregnant	schwanger
baby scales	Babywaage
napkin, nappy (BE), diaper (AE)	Windel
cotton swab, cotton-tipped stick	Wattestäbchen
bath thermometer	Badethermometer
sterilizing tablet	Sterilisiertablette
feeding bottle	Babyflasche
bottle warmer	Fläschchenwärmer
teat (BE), nipple (AE)	Sauger (für Babyflasche)
formula	Milchpulver (der Muttermilch angeglichen)
dummy (BE), pacifier (AE)	Schnuller, Beruhigungssauger
scissors	Schere
blunt	stumpf
lactose	Milchzucker
breastfeed	stillen
baby food	Babynahrung
egg	Ei
noodle	Nudel
rice	Reis
cream	hier: Sahne
spice	Gewürz
onion	Zwiebel
broth	Fleischbrühe
vegetable oil	Pflanzenöl
pork	Schweinefleisch
veal	Kalbfleisch
beef	Rindfleisch
chicken	Huhn
turkey	Pute
celery	Sellerie
potato	Kartoffel
tomato	Tomate
pea	Erbse
carrot	Karotte
puree	Brei
apple	Apfel
banana	Banane
apricot	Aprikose
wholemeal cereals	Vollkorngetreide
powdered	in Pulverform
oatmeal	Haferschrot, Hafermehl
wheat	Weizen
corn	Getreide, Mais
semolina	Grieß
powdered milk	Milchpulver
nut	Nuss
honey	Honig
vitamins	Vitamine
mineral substances	Mineralstoffe
diet	Speiseplan
porridge	Haferbrei
boil	kochen
stir	rühren
fruit juice	Fruchtsaft
fennel	Fenchel
rose-hip	Hagebutte
peppermint	Pfefferminze
camomile	Kamille
orange	Orange
pear	Birne

First aid

first aid	erste Hilfe
accident	Unfall
cause of death	Todesursache
motor vehicle accident	Autounfall
victim	Opfer
knowledge	Kenntnis
first aid kit	Erste-Hilfe-Ausrüstung
accessible	zugänglich
portable	tragbar
unlocked	unverschlossen
reach	Reichweite
label	beschriften
dressing	Verband

wrap	einpacken
safety pin	Sicherheitsnadel
tweezers	Pinzette
cotton wool	Watte
antiseptic	Antiseptikum
sterile	steril
gauze dressing	Mullkompresse
triangular bandage	Dreiecktuch
disposable gloves	Einmalhandschuhe
gauze bandage	Mullbinde
crepe bandage, elastic bandage	elastische Binde
cotton bandage	Baumwollverband
bandage clip	Verbandklammer
waterproof	wasserdicht
adhesive dressing, sticking plaster, adhesive plaster	Wundpflaster
adhesive strapping	Leukoplast

Beauty care and personal hygiene

beauty care	Schönheitspflege
chemist	Apotheker
chemist's shop	Apotheke
expect	erwarten
receive	erhalten
quality	Qualität
advertisement	Reklame
winner	Gewinner
remarkable	bemerkenswert
line	hier: Produktserie
cosmetic	Schönheitspflegeartikel
masculine	männlich
fragrance, scent	Duft
refresh	erfrischen
bold	kühn
unpleasant	unangenehm
shave	Rasur
blend with	mischen mit
odour	Geruch
sunbathe	sonnenbaden
suntan	Sonnenbräune
fall asleep – fell – fallen	einschlafen
soreness	Schmerz, Wundsein
moisture	Feuchtigkeit
intake	Aufnahme
moisturize	Feuchtigkeit verleihen
breath	Atem
mouthwash	Mundwasser
rinse	spülen
care	Pflege
refreshing	erfrischend
toothpaste	Zahnpasta
flavour	Geschmack verleihen
ingredients	Inhaltsstoffe
toothbrush	Zahnbürste
scientific	wissenschaftlich
research	Forschung
beauty	Schönheit
allantoin	Allantoin
promote	fördern
regeneration	Erneuerung
cell	Zelle
irritation of the skin	Hautreizung
hormone	Hormon
sufficient	ausreichend
amount	Menge
cleanse	reinigen
firm	festigen
nourish	nähren, pflegen
thorough	gründlich
dust	Staub
impurity	Unreinheit
instructions for use	Gebrauchsanweisung
apply	auftragen, anwenden, anlegen
tissue	Gewebe, hier: Papiertuch
cotton wool	Watte

facial lotion	Gesichtswasser
render	hier: machen
resistant	widerstandsfähig
moist	feucht
smooth	hier: auftragen
nourishing	Ernährung
texture	Beschaffenheit
radiant	strahlend
fingertip	Fingerspitze

Chapter four

Part one

Conversations at the chemist's

prescription	Rezept
take a seat	Platz nehmen
prepare	zubereiten, vorbereiten
wide	breit
prescribe	verschreiben
make up s. th.	hier: zusammenstellen
recommend	empfehlen
weak	schwach
indicate	angeben, anzeigen
repeat	wiederholen
consult a doctor, go to a doctor, see a doctor	zum Arzt gehen
necessary	notwendig
dentist	Zahnarzt
oculist	Augenarzt
health insurance	Krankenversicherung
insurance company	Versicherungsgesell-schaft
to be employed	angestellt sein
order	bestellen
pharmacy, dispensary	Apotheke
take care of	achtgeben auf
recover	erholen
speedy recovery	gute Besserung

Part two

The chemist's instructions

keep	hier: aufbewahren
tightly closed	dicht verschlossen
away from light, out of direct sunlight	vor Licht geschützt
out of children's reach, out of reach of children	außerhalb der Reichweite von Kindern
keep in a cool place	kühl aufbewahren
fridge, refrigerator	Kühlschrank
deepfreezer	Tiefkühlfach, -truhe
highly inflammable	leicht entzündlich
external	äußerlich
internal	innerlich
not to be taken	nicht einnehmen
toxic	toxisch
inhale	einatmen
swallow	schlucken
mucous membrane	Schleimhaut
danger	Gefahr
poison	Gift
dose	Dosis
exceed	übersteigen
in the absence of specific instructions from your doctor	falls vom Arzt nicht anders verordnet
before breakfast	auf nüchternen Magen
chew	kauen
swallow	hinunterschlucken
dissolve	auflösen
liquid	Flüssigkeit
suck	lutschen
let ... melt	zergehen lassen
shake – shook – shaken	schütteln
undiluted	unverdünnt
a tablespoonful of cold water	ein Esslöffel Wasser
rinse	spülen

measuring spoonful	Messlöffel
corn	Hühnerauge
complete bath	Vollbad
hip bath	Sitzbad
remove wrapping	Verpackung, Umhüllung entfernen
insert	einführen
apply	hier: auftragen
rub (in)	(ein)reiben
lay on	auflegen
cover	bedecken
dress	verbinden
apply a bandage	einen Verband anlegen
leave ... open	... offen lassen
minute	winzig
sprinkle	streuen
sip	in kleinen Schlucken trinken
three teaspoonfuls	drei Teelöffel
mix	mischen
boil	kochen
steep	(den Tee) ziehen lassen
instant tea	löslicher Tee
saw	Säge

Chapter five

Exercises

wet	nass
perm(anent wave)	Dauerwelle
hairdryer	Haartrockner
curling pin	Lockenstab
roller	Lockenwickler
iodine	Jod
practice	Praxis
consulting hours	Sprechstunde
inflammable	entzündlich
relief	Erleichterung
nursing home	Pflegeheim
to shake – shook – shaken	schütteln
to mix	mischen
habit	Gewohnheit
to recommend	empfehlen
circulation	Kreislauf
excess	Übermaß
cut	Schnitt
graze	Schürfwunde
breakfast	Frühstück
at bedtime	vor dem Zubettgehen
meal	Mahlzeit
scalp	Kopfhaut
limp	schlaff
graesy	fettig
itchy	juckend
tight	gespannt
comfortable	angenehm
to improve	verbessern
shine	Glanz
coarse	rau
brittle	brüchig
comb	Kamm
split ends	gespaltene Spitzen

7.2. Alphabetical word list German – English

BE = British English
AE = American English
coll. = colloquial (Umgangssprache)

Abführmittel	laxative
abhängig werden von	get addicted to
absondern	secrete
absorbieren	absorb
Abszess	abscess
Achsel	armpit
achtgeben auf	to take care of
After	anus
Allantoin	allantoin
Allergie	allergy
allergisch	allergic

Allgemeinmediziner	general practitioner
Alter	age
ambulante(r) Patient(in)	outpatient
Ampulle	ampoule, ampule
angeboren	inborn
angenehm	comfortable
Angina Pectoris	angina pectoris
Angst haben	to be afraid (of)
Anis	anise
sich anstecken	to catch
Antiseptikum	antiseptic
Anweisung	instruction
Anwendung	application, administration
Apotheke	chemist's (shop), dispensary, pharmacy, drugstore (AE)
Apotheker	chemist, dispenser, pharmacist, druggist (AE)
Arm	arm
Arnika	arnica
Arterie	artery
Arzneibuch	pharmacopoeia
Arzneimittel	medicine, remedy, medicament
Arzneimittel, Rauschgift	drug
ein Arzneimitel gegen etw.	a remedy for s. th.
Arzt	doctor, physician
zum Arzt gehen	to consult a doctor, to go to a doctor, to see a doctor
Asthma	asthma
Atem	breath
Atemnot	difficulty in breathing
auflösen	to dissolve
auftragen, anwenden (z. B. Salbe)	to apply
auftreten	to arise – arose – arisen

Auge	eye
Augenarzt	oculist
Augenbad	eye solution
Augenbraue	eyebrow
Augenhöhle	socket of the eye
Augenlid	eyelid
Augensalbe	eye ointment
Augentropfen	eye drops
Augenwinkel	corner of the eye
Ausgesetztsein	exposure
Ausschlag	rash, eruption
außerhalb der Reichweite von Kindern	out of children's reach, ... reach of children
Babyflasche	feeding bottle
Babynahrung	baby food
Babywaage	baby scales
Badethermometer	bath thermometer
Bakterie(n)	bacterium, bacteria
Baldrian	valerian
Balsam	balsam
Band	ligament
Bärlapp	club-moss
Bart	beard
Bauch	abdomen, belly
Bauchschmerzen	abdominal pains, stomachache
Bauchspeicheldrüse	pancreas
Baumwollverband	cotton bandage
befallen, betreffen	to affect
behandeln	to treat
Beifuß	mugwort
Bein	leg
beißen	to bite – bit – bitten
Beruhigungsmittel	sedative, tranquillizer
beschriften	to label
Beschwerde	complaint
Bestandteil	constituent
bestehen aus	to consist of
bestellen	to order
Beweglichkeit	flexibility

Bewusstlosigkeit	unconsciousness
Bewusstsein	consciousness
Birke	birch
Blase (auf der Haut)	blister
(Harn)blase	bladder
Blasenwerfen	blistering
blass	pale
blauer Fleck, Quetschung	bruise
blind	blind
Blinddarm	appendix
Blinddarm-entzündung	appendicitis
Blut	blood
Blutdruck	blood pressure
Blutfette	blood fats
Blutfettwerte	plasma lipid concentration
Blutgefäß	blood vessel
Blutgerinnsel	blood clot
Blutkreislauf	blood circulation
Blutzufuhr	blood supply
Bonbon	(medical) toffee
bösartig (Tumor)	malignant
Brandbinde	bismuth bandage for burns
Brandwunde	burn
Brausegranulat	effervescent granules
Brausetabletten	effervescent tablets
brechen	to break – broke – broken
Brechwurzel, Ipecacuanha	ipecac
breit	wide
Brennessel	stinging nettle
Brille	glasses
Brombeere	blackberry
Bronchien	bronchi, bronchial tubes
Bronchitis	bronchitis
Broschüre, Merkblatt	leaflet
brüchig	brittle

Brust	breast
Brustbein	breastbone
Brustkorb	chest
Brustwarze	nipple
Celsius	centigrade
Chirurg	surgeon
Cholera	cholera
Cholesterinspiegel	cholesterol level
Creme	cream
Darm	intestine(s), bowel(s)
Dauerwelle	perm(anent wave)
Daumen	thumb
Diabetes	diabetes
dick	thick
Dickdarm	great gut, large intestine, colon
Dienstag	Tuesday
Dilution	Dilution
Diphtherie	diphtheria
Donnerstag	Thursday
Dosier-Aerosol	aerosol
Dosis	dose
Dragée	coated tablet, dragee
Dreiecktuch	triangular bandage
Druckknopf	press stud, popper
Drüse	gland
Drüsenflüssigkeit	glandular liquid
Duft	fragrance, scent
dünn	thin
Dünndarm	small gut, small intestine
Durchfall	diarrhoea
Efeu	ivy
Eibisch	marshmallow
einatmen	inhale
einführen	insert
Einlauf	enema
einpacken	to wrap
(ein)reiben	to rub (in)
Einreibung	inunction

Eiter	matter, pus
eitern	to fester
Eiterung	suppuration
elastische Binde	crepe bandage, elastic bandage
Ellbogen	elbow
Elle	ulna
Embolie	embolism
empfehlen	to recommend
empfindlich	sensitive
Emulsion	emulsion
enthalten	to contain
leicht entzündlich	highly inflammable
Enthaarungscreme	depilatory cream
entzündlich	inflammable
Entzündung	inflammation
Enzian	gentian
epidemisch, Epidemie	epidemic
Epilepsie	epilepsy
erbrechen	to vomit
Erdbeere	strawberry
erfrischen	to refresh
erfrischend	refreshing
erholen	to recover
Erkältung	cold
eine Erkältung bekommen	to catch a cold
erklären	to explain
Erleichterung	relief
Erröten	reddening
erste Hilfe	first aid
Erste-Hilfe-Ausrüstung	first aid kit
Esslöffel	tablespoon
zwei Esslöffel	two tablespoonfuls
Eukalyptus	eucalyptus
Extrakt	extract
(Cholera)fall	case (of cholera)
Falte	wrinkle
Fenchel	fennel
Ferse	heel
Fett	fat
fettig	greasy
Fettpolster	pads of fat
Fettsalbe	greasy ointment
Fieber	fever
Finger	finger
kleiner Finger	little finger
Fingernagel	fingernail
Fingerspitze	fingertip
Fläschchenwärmer	bottle warmer
Fleck	spot
Fleckfieber	typhus
Flüssigkeit	fluid, liquid
Forschung	research
Frauenarzt	gynaecologist
Freitag	Friday
Fruchtsaft	fruit juice
Frühstück	breakfast
Fuß	foot – feet
Fußknöchel	ankle
Galle	bile
Gallenblase	gall bladder
Gallensteine	gall stones
Gänsehaut	goose pimples
Gaumen	palate
Gaumenzäpfchen	uvula
Gebrauchsanweisung	instructions for use
gebrauchsfertig	ready for use
Gebrechen, Leiden	ailment
Geburt	(child)birth
Gehirn	brain
Gehirnerschütterung	concussion of the brain
geistig, seelisch	mental
Gel	gel
Gelbfieber	yellow fever
Gelbsucht, Hepatitis	hepatitis
Gelbwurz	tumeric
Gelenk	joint
gerötet	flushed
Geruch	odour
Geruchsorgan	organ of smell

Gesäß	buttocks
Geschlechts- krankheit	venereal disease, V. D.
Geschmacksknospen	taste buds
Geschmackssinn	sense of taste
Geschwür	ulcer
Gesicht	face
Gesichtsfarbe	complexion
Gesichtswasser	facial lotion
gespaltene Spitzen	split ends
gespannt	tight
gesund	healthy
Gesundheit	health
Gesundheitsproblem	health problem
Gewebe	tissue
Gewohnheit	habit
Gift	poison
giftig	poisonous, toxic
Ginster	broom
Glanz	shine
glattrasiert	cleanshaven
Gleichgewichtsorgan	organ of balance
Gliedmaßen	limbs
... Grad Celsius	... degrees centigrade
Granulat	granules
Grippe	influenza, flu
Grund	reason
Gurgelmittel	gargle
gut verschlossen	tightly closed
gutartig (Tumor)	benign
gute Besserung	speedy recovery
Haar(e)	hair
Haaransatz	hair-line
Haartrockner	hairdryer
Hafer	oats (Pl.)
Hagebutte	rose-hip
Hals	neck
Hals, Rachen	throat
Hämorrhoiden	haemorrhoids, piles
Hand	hand
Handgelenk	wrist
Hanf	hemp
Hart(gelatine)kapseln	hard gelatine capsule
Haut	skin
Hautabschürfung	skin abrasion
Hautarzt	dermatologist
Hautreizungen	irritations of the skin
Heftpflaster, Leukoplast	adhesive strapping, first aid tape
Heidelbeere	blueberry
heilen	to cure
Heilmittel s. Arzneimittel	
Heiserkeit	hoarseness
Herbstzeitlose	meadow saffron
Herz	heart
Herz- und Gefäß-...	cardiovascular
Herzanfall	heart attack
Herzbeklemmungen	constriction of the heart
Herzbeschwerden	heart complaints
Herzfehler	heart defect
Herzinfarkt	cardiac infarction
Herzinsuffizienz	cardiac insufficiency
Herzprobleme	hearttrouble
Herzrhythmus	heart rhythm
Herzschlag	heartbeat
Herzstillstand	heart arrest
Herzversagen	heart failure
Hexenschuss	lumbago
Himbeere	raspberry
Hirnhautentzündung	meningitis
Hitzschlag	heatstroke
Holunder	elder
homöopathische Lösungen	homeopathic solutions
Hopfen	hop
Hormon	hormone
Huflattich	coltsfoot
Hüfte	hip
Hüftknochen	hip-bone
Hühnerauge	corn
Husten	cough

husten	to cough
Hustensaft	cough mixture, cough syrup
Hustentropfen	cough drops
Hygiene	hygiene
Impfung	vaccination
Infektion	infection
Infektionskrankheit	infectious disease
Infusionslösung	infusion
Ingwer	ginger
Injektionsflasche	vial
Injektionslösung	injection
Inhalationslösung	inhalation solution
Inhaltsstoffe	ingredients
Inkubationszeit	incubation period
Innenohr	inner ear
inneres Organ	internal organ
innerlich	internal(ly)
Insulin	insulin
Iod	iodine
Iris	iris
Ischias	sciatica
Jod	iodine
juckend	itchy
Kamille	camomile
Kamm	comb
Kapsel	capsule
Kardamom	cardamom
Kartoffel	potato
kauen	to chew
Kautabletten	chewing tablets
Keim, Bazillus	germ
Keuchhusten	whooping cough, pertussis
Kiefer	jaw
Kind, Kinder	child, children
Kinderarzt	paediatrician
Kinderlähmung	polio(myelitis)
Kinn	chin
Kirsche	cherry
Klistier	enema
Klysma	enema
Knie	knee
Kniescheibe	knee-cap
Knochen	bone
Knochenbruch	fracture
Knochenmark	bone-marrow
kochen	to boil
Kohlehydrat	carbohydrate
Kohletablette	charcoal tablet
Kolik	colic
Koordinations-zentrum	coordinating centre
Kopf	head
Kopfhaut	scalp
Kopfschmerzen	headache
Kornblume	cornflower
Körper	body
Körperteil	part of the body
Körpertemperatur	body temperature
Krampf	cramp
Krampfadern	varicose veins
krank	ill (präd.), sick (attrib.)
Krankenhaus	hospital
Krankenschwester	nurse
Krankenversicherung	health insurance
Krankheit	illness, disease, sickness
Krebs	cancer
Kreislauf	circulation
Kreislauf-	circulatory
kühl aufbewahren	keep in a cool place
Kühlschrank	refrigerator, fridge
Kümmel	caraway
Kummer, Herzeleid	heartache
Kunde	customer
Kurort	spa
kurzsichtig	short-sighted
Lähmung	paralysis
Lavendel	lavender
Leber	liver

leiden an	to suffer from
Leinsamen	linseed
Leiste	groin
Leukämie	leukemia
Liebstöckl	lovage
Linde	lime tree
Liniment	Liniment
Lippe	lip
Lockenstab	curling pin
Lockenwickler	roller
lockig	curly
Lorbeer	laurel
löslicher Tee	instant tea
Lösung	solution
Lotion	lotion
Löwenzahn	dandelion
Luftröhre	windpipe
Lunge	lung(s)
Lungenentzündung	pneumonia
lutschen	to suck
Lymphgewebe	lymphoid tissue
Magen	stomach, tummy
Magenverstimmung	indigestion
Mahlzeit	meal
Maiglöckchen	lily of the valley
Majoran	majoram
Malaria	malaria
Malve	mallow
Mandelentzündung	tonsillitis
Mandeln	tonsils
männlich	masculine
Masern	measles
Medikament s. Arzneimittel	
medizinisch	medical
Melisse	melissa
menschlich	human
Menstruations-beschwerden	period pains
Messlöffel	measuring spoonful
Migräne	migraine
Milch	milk
Milchpulver	powdered milk
Milchpulver (der Muttermilch angeglichen)	formula
Milchzucker	lactose
Milz	spleen
Mineralstoffe	mineral substances
mischen	to mix
Mistel	mistletoe
Mittelfinger	middle finger
Mittwoch	Wednesday
Mixtur	mixture
Mohn	poppy
Montag	Monday
müde	tired
Müdigkeit, Mattigkeit	weariness
Mullbinde	gauze bandage
Mullkompresse	gauze dressing
Mumps	mumps
Mund	mouth
Mundwasser	mouthwash
Muskatnuss	nutmeg
Muskel	muscle
Muskelfaserriss	rupture of a muscle fibre
Muttermal	birthmark
Myrrhe	myrrh
Nabel	navel
nähren, pflegen	to nourish
Nase	nose
Nasenbein	nasal bone
Nasenbluten	nosebleed
Nasengel	nose gel
Nasenhöhle	nasal cavity
Nasenloch	nostril
Nasensalbe	nose ointment
Nasenspray	nose spray
Nasentropfen	nose drops
nass	wet
Nebenwirkung	side effects

Nervensystem	nervous system
Neurologe	neurologist
nicht einnehmen	not to be taken
Niere	kidney
Nierenentzündung	nephritis
niesen	to sneeze
nüchtern, auf nüchternen Magen	not having breakfasted, before having eaten anything
Oberarm	upper arm
Oberschenkel	thigh
in Ohnmacht fallen	to faint
Ohr	ear
Ohrentropfen	ear drops
ölig	lubricant
Operation	operation
etw. operieren	to operate on s. th.
Organ	organ
Orthopäde	orthopaedist
Paste	paste
Pastille	lozenge
Patient	patient
Pfeffer	pepper
Pfefferminze	peppermint
Pfeiffersches Drüsenfieber	mononucleosis
Pflegeheim	nursing home
Pflaster	plaster
Pflege	care, nursing
Pharmakologie	pharmacology
Pickel	pimple
Pinzette	tweezers
Plattfüße	flat feet
Platz nehmen	to take a seat
Pocken	smallpox
Pollen	pollen
Polypen	adenoids
praktischer Arzt	G. P., general practitioner
Praxis	practice

Psychiater	psychiatrist
psychiatrische Behandlung	psychiatric treatment
Pubertät	puberty
Pulver, Puder	powder
in Pulverform	powdered
Pulvermischungen	powder mixture
Pulvertee	powdered tea
Pupille	pupil
Rasur	shave
Rat	advice
rau	coarse
rauchen	to smoke
Regulierung	regulation
Rektalsalbe	rectal ointment
reinigen	to cleanse
Reiseübelkeit	travel-sickness
reißen	to tear – tore – torn
Reklame	advertisement
Retardkapseln	retardation capsules
Rezept	prescription
Rhabarber	rhubarb
Rheumatismus	rheumatism
Rindfleisch	beef
Ringelblume	marigold
Ringfinger	ring finger, third finger
Rippe	rib
Risikofaktor	risk factor
Roggen	rye
Rollstuhl	wheelchair
Röntgenabteilung	x-ray department
Rose	rose
Rosmarin	rosemary
Rosskastanie	horse chestnut
Röteln	German measles
Rücken	back
Rückenschmerzen	backache
Ruhr	dysentery
rühren	to stir
Rumpf	trunk

Safran, Crocus	saffron
Saft	juice
Säge	saw
Salbe	ointment
Salbei	sage
Samstag	Saturday
Sauger (für Babyflasche)	teat (BE), nipple (AE)
Säuglingspflege	baby care
Schachtelhalm, Zinnkraut	horsetail
Schädel	skull
Schafgarbe	yarrow
Scharlach	scarlet fever
Scheitel	parting
Schere	scissors
Schienbein	shin, shinbone, tibia
Schilddrüse	thyroid (gland)
Schläfe	temple
schlaff	limp
Schlaflosigkeit	sleeplessness, insomnia
Schlaftablette	sleeping pill, tablets for insomnia
Schlag(anfall)	stroke (coll.)
Schlaganfall	apoplectic fit
Schleim	mucus
Schleimhaut	mucous membrane
schlucken	to swallow
in kleinen Schlucken trinken	to sip
etw. ganz hinunterschlucken	to swallow s. th. whole
Schlüsselblume, Primel	cowslip
schmecken	to taste
Schmerz, Wundsein	soreness
schmerzen	to ache
schmerzhaft	painful
Schmerzmittel	pain-killer, anodyne
Schnitt	cut
Schnuller	dummy (BE), pacifier (AE)
Schnupfen	catarrh
Schnurrbart	moustache
Schönheitspflege	beautycare
Schönheitspflegeartikel	cosmetic
Schulter	shoulder
Schulterblatt	shoulder-blade
Schürfwunde	graze
Schüttelfrost	shivering fit
schütteln	to shake – shook – shaken
schützen	to protect
schwach	weak
schwanger	pregnant
Schwangerschaft	pregnancy
schwellen	to swell – swelled – swollen
Schwertlilie	Iris
schwindelig	dizzy
schwitzen	to sweat
Seekrankheit	sea-sickness
Sehne	sinew, tendon
Sehnenscheiden-entzündung	inflammation of the tendon sheath
Seitenstechen	stitches in the side
Sennespflanze	senna
sich Sorgen machen	to worry
Sicherheitsnadel	safety pin
Sirup	syrup
Sitzbad	hip bath
Skelett, Knochengerüst	skeleton
Sodbrennen	heartburn
Sohle	sole
Sommersprossen	freckles
sonnenbaden	to sunbathe
Sonnenbrand	sunburn
Sonnenbräune	suntan
Sonnenstich	sunstroke
Sonntag	Sunday
Speiche	radius
Speiseplan	diet
Speiseröhre	gullet
Spray	spray

sprechen	to speak
Sprechstunde	consulting hours
Spreizfüße	splay feet
spülen	to rinse
Spüllösung	washing
Stärke	starch
stechen	to sting – stung – stung
Steifheit	stiffness
Steingefäß, Krug	jar
sterben (an)	to die (from, of)
steril	sterile
Sterilisiertablette	sterilizing tablet
stillen	to breastfeed, -fed, -fed
Stirn	forehead
Stirnhöhlen	sinuses
Stirnhöhlenkatarrh	sinusitis
Störung	disorder
Stoffwechsel	metabolism
streuen	to sprinkle
stumm	mute
stumpf	blunt
Sublingualtablette	sublingual tablet
Suspension	suspension
Süßholzwurzel	liquorice root
Symptom	symptom
Tablette	tablet
Taille	waist
Tang	seaweed
taub	deaf
Taubnessel	deadnettle
taubstumm	deaf and dumb
Tee	tea
Teeaufgussbeutel	teabag
Teelöffel	teaspoonful
Temperatur	temperature
eine hohe Temperatur haben	to run a high temperature
Thermometer	thermometer
Thrombose(n)	thrombosis (thromboses)
Thymian	thyme
Tinktur	tincture
Tod	death
Todesursache	cause of death
tödlich	killing
Tollkirsche, Belladonna	deadly night shade
toxisch	toxic
Trommelfell	eardrum
Tropfen	drops
tropisch	tropical
Tuberkulose	tuberculosis
Tumor, Geschwulst	tumour
Typhus	typhoid (fever)
Übelkeit	nausea, sickness
übergewichtig	overweight
Übermaß	excess
im Übermaß nehmen	to take to excess
unerlässlich	essential
Unfall	accident
unregelmäßig	irregular
Unterarm	forearm
untersuchen	to examine
unverdünnt	undiluted
Vaginalcreme	vaginal cream
Vaginalzäpfchen	vaginal suppositories
Vene	vein
ver-, ausrenken	to dislocate
Verband	dressing, bandage
einen Verband anlegen	to apply a bandage
Verbandklammer	bandage clip
verbessern	to improve
eine Wunde verbinden	to dress a wound
verdauen	to digest
Verdauungskanal	alimentary canal
Verdauungsstörung	indigestion
Verdauungssystem	digestive system
Verdauungstrakt	digestive tract
verletzen	to injure, to hurt
Verletzung	injury

Verordnung, Medikamente	medication
Verpackung	wrapping
verschreiben	to prescribe
verschreibungsfreies Medikament	OTC-drug
verschreibungs-pflichtiges Medikament	ethical
Versicherung(s-gesellschaft)	insurance company
verstauchen	to sprain
Verstopfung	constipation
Virus	virus
Virus-	viral
Vitamin	vitamin
Vollbad	complete bath
Vollkorngetreide	wholemeal cereals
vor Licht geschützt	out of direct sunlight, away from light
vorbeugend, Prophylaktikum	prophylactic
Vorsichtsmaßnahme	precaution
Wacholder	juniper
wachsen	to grow – grew – grown
Wade	calf – calves
Wadenbein	fibula
Waldmeister	woodruff
Walnuss	walnut
Wange	cheek
Warze	wart
wasserdicht	waterproof
wässrig	aqueous
Watte	cotton wool (BE), cotton (AE)
Wattestäbchen	cotton swab, cotton-tipped sticks, cotton bud
Wegerich	plantain
weiblich/männlich	female/male
Weich(gelatine)kapseln	soft gelatine capsules
Weide	willow
Weißdorn	hawthorn
weitsichtig	long-sighted, far-sighted
Weizen	wheat
Wermut	wormwood
Wermut-Wein	vermouth
wesentlich	essential
widerstandsfähig	resistant
Wimpern	eyelashes
Windel	napkin, nappy (BE), diaper (AE)
Windpocken	chickenpox
Wirbel	vertebra
Wirbelsäule	vertebral column, backbone, spine
wissenschaftlich	scientific
wund	sore
Wundbenzin	surgical spirit
Wundpflaster	adhesive dressing, adhesive plaster, elastoplast, sticking plaster, first aid tape
Wundstarrkrampf	tetanus
Zahn – Zähne	tooth – teeth
Zahnarzt	dentist
Zahnbürste	toothbrush
Zahnfleisch	gum
Zahnpasta	toothpaste
Zahnschmerzen	toothache
Zäpfchen	suppository
Zehe	toe
Zeichen	sign
Zeigefinger	forefinger, index finger
Zelle	cell
Zellteilung	cell division
zergehen lassen	to let ... melt
zerren	to strain
(den Tee) ziehen lassen	steep
Zigarettenrauchen	cigarette smoking
Zimt	cinnamon
Zitronenbaum	lemon tree

zittern	to shiver
zubereiten, vorbereiten	to prepare
vor dem Zubettgehen	at bedtime
Zuckerspiegel	sugar content
Zunge	tongue
zusammengesetzt aus	composed of
Zwiebel	onion

7.3. Alphabetical word list English – German

a remedy for	ein Medikament gegen
abdomen	Bauch
abdominal pains	Bauchschmerzen
abscess	Abszess
absorb	absorbieren
accident	Unfall
ache	schmerzen
aconite	Eisenhut
adenoids	Polypen
adhesive dressing	Wundpflaster
adhesive plaster	Wundpflaster
adhesive strapping	Leukoplast, Heftpflaster
administration	Anwendung
advertisement	Reklame
advice	Rat
aerosol	Aerosol, Dosierspray
affect	befallen, betreffen, angreifen
afraid (of)	Angst haben
age	Alter
ailment	Gebrechen, Leiden
alimentary canal	Verdauungskanal
allantoin	Allantoin
allergic	allergisch
allergy	Allergie
ampoule, ampule	Ampulle
angina pectoris	Angina pectoris
anise	Anis
ankle	Fußknöchel
anodyne	Schmerzmittel
antiseptic	Antiseptikum
anus	After
apoplectic fit	Schlaganfall
appendicitis	Blinddarm-entzündung
appendix	Blinddarm
application	Anwendung
apply	auftragen, anwenden, anlegen
apply a bandage	einen Verband anlegen
aqueous	wässrig
arise – arose – arisen	auftreten
arm	Arm
armpit	Achsel
arnica	Arnika
artery	Arterie
asthma	Asthma
at bedtime	vor dem Zubettgehen
away from light	vor Licht geschützt
baby scales	Babywaage
baby care	Säuglingspflege
baby food	Babynahrung
back	Rücken
backache	Rückenschmerzen
backbone	Wirbelsäule
bacterium, bacteria	Bakterie(n)
bald	kahlköpfig
balsam	Balsam
bandage clip	Verbandklammer
bandaid	Wundpflaster
bath thermometer	Badethermometer
beard	Bart
beauty care	Schönheitspflege
beef	Rindfleisch
before having eaten anything, before breakfast	nüchtern, auf nüchternen Magen

belly	Bauch
benign	gutartig
bile	Galle
birch	Birke
birth	Geburt
birthmark	Muttermal
bismuth bandage for burns	Brandbinde
bite – bit – bitten	beißen
blackberry	Brombeere
bladder	Blase
blind	blind
blood clot	Blutgerinnsel
blood supply	Blutzufuhr
body temperature	Körpertemperatur
boil	kochen
bone	Knochen
bone-marrow	Knochenmark
bottle warmer	Fläschchenwärmer
bowel(s)	Darm
brain	Gehirn
break – broke – broken	brechen
breakfast	Frühstück
breast	Brust
breastbone	Brustbein
breastfeed – -fed – -fed	stillen
breath	Atem
brittle	brüchig
bronchial tubes, bronchi	Bronchien
bronchitis	Bronchitis
broom	Ginster
bruise	blauer Fleck, Quetschung
burn	Brandwunde
buttocks	Gesäß
calf – calves	Wade
camomile	Kamille
cancer	Krebs
capsule	Kapsel
caraway	Kümmel
carbohydrate	Kohlehydrat
cardamom	Kardamom
cardiac infarction	Herzinfarkt
cardiac insufficiency	Herzinsuffizienz
cardiovascular	Herz- und Gefäß
care	Pflege
case (of cholera)	(Cholera)fall
catarrh	Schnupfen
catch	sich anstecken
catch a cold	eine Erkältung bekommen
cause of death	Todesursache
cell	Zelle
cell division	Zellteilung
centigrade	Celsius
charcoal tablet	Kohletablette
cheek	Wange
chemist	Apotheker
chemist's (shop)	Apotheke
cherry	Kirsche
chest	Brustkorb
chew	kauen
chewing tablets	Kautabletten
chicken pox	Windpocken
child, children	Kind, Kinder
childbirth	Geburt
chin	Kinn
cholera	Cholera
cholesterol level	Cholesterinspiegel
cigarette smoking	Zigarettenrauchen
cinnamon	Zimt
circulation	Kreislauf
circulatory	Kreislauf-
cirrhosis of liver	Leber-zirrhose
cleanse	reinigen
cleanshaven	glattrasiert
club-moss	Bärlapp
coarse	rau
coated tablet, dragée	Dragée

cold	Erkältung
colic	Kolik
colon	Dickdarm
coltsfoot	Huflattich
comb	Kamm
combination pack:	Kombipackung
ointment	= Salbe
+ suppositories	+ Zäpfchen
comfortable	angenehm
complaints	Beschwerden
complete bath	Vollbad
complexion	Gesichtsfarbe
component	Bestandteil
concussion	
of the brain	Gehirnerschütterung
consciousness	Bewusstsein
consist of	bestehen aus
constipation	Verstopfung
constituent	Bestandteil
constriction	Herz-
ot the heart	beklemmungen
consult a doctor	zum Arzt gehen
consulting hours	Sprechstunde
contain	enthalten
coordinating centre	Koordinationszentrum
corn	Hühnerauge, Mais
corner of the eye	Augenwinkel
cornflower	Kornblume
cosmetic	Schönheitspflegeartikel
cotton (AE)	Watte
cotton bandage	Baumwollverband
cotton bud	Wattestäbchen
cotton swab	Wattestäbchen
cotton wool (BE)	Watte
cotton-tipped sticks	Wattestäbchen
cough	Husten
cough	husten
cough drops	Hustentropfen
cough mixture	Hustensaft
cowslip	Schlüsselblume
cramp	Krampf
cream	Creme
crepe bandage	elastische Binde
cure	heilen
curling pin	Lockenstab
curly	lockig
customer	Kunde
cut	Schnitt
dandelion	Löwenzahn
deadly nightshade	Tollkirsche, Belladonna
deadnettle	Taubnessel
deaf	taub
deaf and dumb	taubstumm
death	Tod
... degrees centigrade	... Grad Celsius
dentist	Zahnarzt
depilatory cream	Enthaarungscreme
dermatologist	Hautarzt
diabetes	Diabetes
diaper (AE)	Windel
diarrhoea	Durchfall
die	sterben
die from/of	sterben an
diet	Speiseplan
difficulty in breathing	Atemnot
digest	verdauen
digestive system	Verdauungssystem
digestive tract	Verdauungstrakt
dilution	Dilution
diphtheria	Diphtherie
disease	Krankheit
dislocate	ver- ausrenken
disorder	Störung
dispensary	Apotheke
dispenser	Apotheker
disposable gloves	Einmalhandschuhe
dissolve	auflösen
dizzy	schwindelig
dose	Dosis
dress (a wound)	verbinden
dressing	Verband
drops	Tropfen
drug	Arzneimittel, Rauschgift

druggist (AE)	Apotheker
drugstore (AE)	Apotheke
dummy (BE)	Schnuller, Beruhigungssauger
dysentery	Ruhr
ear	Ohr
eardrum	Trommelfell
eardrops	Ohrentropfen
effervescent granules	Brausegranulat
effervescent tablet	Brausetabletten
elastic bandage	elastische Binde
elastoplast	Wundpflaster
elbow	Ellbogen
elder	Holunder
embolism	Embolie
embrocation	Einreibung
emulsion	Emulsion
enema	Klysma = Einlauf = Klistier
epidemic	epidemisch, Epidemie
epilepsy	Epilepsie
eruption	Hautausschlag
essential	wesentlich, unerlässlich
ethical	verschreibungspflichtiges Medikament
eucalyptus	Eukalyptus
examine	untersuchen
excess	Übermaß
explain	erklären
exposure	Ausgesetztsein
external	äußerlich
extract	Extrakt
eye	Auge
eyeball	Augapfel
eye ointment	Augensalbe
eyesocket	Augenhöhle
eye solution	Augenbad
eyebrow	Augenbraue
eyedrops	Augentropfen
eyelashes	Wimpern
eyelid	Augenlid
face	Gesicht
facial lotion	Gesichtswasser
faint	in Ohnmacht fallen
far-sighted	weitsichtig
fat	Fett
feeding bottle	Babyflasche
female/male	weiblich/männlich
fennel	Fenchel
fester	eitern
fever	Fieber
fibula	Wadenbein
finger	Finger
fingernail	Fingernagel
fingertip	Fingerspitze
first aid	erste Hilfe
first aid kit	Erste-Hilfe-Ausrüstung
first aid tape	Leukoplast, Heftpflaster
flat feet	Plattfüße
flexibility	Beweglichkeit
flu (influenza)	Grippe
fluid	Flüssigkeit
flushed	gerötet
foot – feet	Fuß – Füße
forearm	Unterarm
forefinger	Zeigefinger
forehead	Stirn
formula	Milchpulver (der Muttermilch angeglichen)
fragrance	Duft
fracture	Knochenbruch
freckles	Sommersprossen
Friday	Freitag
fridge	Kühlschrank
fruit juice	Fruchtsaft
G. P. see general practitioner	

gall bladder	Gallenblase
gall stones	Gallensteine
gargle	Gurgelmittel
gauze bandage	Mullbinde
gauze dressing	Mullkompresse
gel	Gel
general practitioner	Allgemeinmediziner
gentian	Enzian
germ	Keim, Bazillus
German measles	Röteln
get addicted to	abhängig werden von
ginger	Ingwer
gland	Drüse, Schilddrüse
glandular liquid	Drüsenflüssigkeit
glasses	Brille
go to the doctor	zum Arzt gehen
goose pimples	Gänsehaut
granules	Granulat
graze	Schürfwunde
greasy	fettig
greasy ointment	Fettsalbe
groin	Leiste
grow – grew – grown	wachsen
gullet	Speiseröhre
gum	Zahnfleisch
gynaecologist	Frauenarzt
habit	Gewohnheit
haemorrhoids	Hämorrhoiden
hair	Haar(e)
hairdryer	Haartrockner
hair-line	Haaransatz
hand	Hand
hard gelatine capsule	Hart(gelatine)kapsel
hawthorn	Weißdorn
head	Kopf
headache	Kopfschmerzen
health	Gesundheit
health insurance	Krankenversicherung
health problem	Gesundheitsproblem
healthy	gesund
heart	Herz
heart arrest	Herzstillstand
heart attack	Herzanfall
heart trouble	Herzbeschwerden
heart defect	Herzfehler
heart failure	Herzversagen
heart rhythm	Herzrhythmus
heartache	Kummer, Herzeleid
heartbeat	Herzschlag
heartburn	Sodbrennen
heatstroke	Hitzschlag
heel	Ferse
hemp	Hanf
hepatitis	Hepatitis, Gelbsucht
herbs	Kräuter
highly inflammable	leicht entzündlich
hip	Hüfte
hip bath	Sitzbad
hip-bone	Hüftknochen
hoarseness	Heiserkeit
homeopathic solution	Homöopathische Lösung
hop	Hopfen
hormone	Hormon
horse chestnut	Roßkastanie
horsetail	Schachtelhalm
hospital	Krankenhaus
hot	heiß
human	menschlich
humane	human, menschlich
hygiene	Hygiene
ill	krank
illness	Krankheit
improve	verbessern
inborn	angeboren
incubation period	Inkubationszeit
index finger	Zeigefinger
indigestion	Verdauungsstörung
infection	Infektion
infectious disease	Infektionskrankheit
inflammation	Entzündung

inflammation of the tendon	Sehnen(scheiden)entzündung
inflammable	entzündlich
influenza	Grippe
infusion	Infusions(lösung)
ingredient	Inhaltsstoff
inhalation	Einatmung
inhalation solution	Inhalationslösung
injection	Injektions(lösung)
injury	Verletzung
inner ear	Innenohr
insert	einführen
insomnia	Schlaflosigkeit
instant tea	löslicher Tee
instruction	Anweisung
instructions for use	Gebrauchsanweisung
insulin	Insulin
insurance company	Versicherung(sgesellschaft)
internal(ly)	innerlich
intestine(s)	Darm
iodine	Jod
ipecac	Brechwurzel
iris	Schwertlilie, Iris
irregular	unregelmäßig
irritation of the skin	Hautreizung
itchy	juckend
ivy	Efeu
jar	Steingefäß, Krug
jaw	Kiefer
joint	Gelenk
juice	(Frucht-)Saft
juniper	Wacholder
keep in a cool place	kühl aufbewahren
kidney	Niere
killing	tödlich
knee	Knie
knee-cap	Kniescheibe
label	beschriften, Etikett
lactose	Milchzucker
large intestine	Dickdarm
laurel	Lorbeer
lavender	Lavendel
laxative	Abführmittel
leaflet	Broschüre, Merkblatt, Beipackzettel
leg	Bein
lemon tree	Zitronenbaum
let ... melt	zergehen lassen
leukemia	Leukämie
ligament	Band
lily of the valley	Maiglöckchen
limbs	Gliedmaßen
lime tree	Linde
limp	schlaff
liniment	Liniment
linseed	Leinsamen
lip	Lippe
liquid	Flüssigkeit
liquorice root	Süßholzwurzel
little finger	kleiner Finger
liver	Leber
long-sighted	weitsichtig
lotion	Lotion
lovage	Liebstöckl
lozenge	Pastille
lubricant	ölig
lumbago	Hexenschuss
lung(s)	Lunge
Lymphoid tissue	Lymphgewebe
majoram	Majoran
malaria	Malaria
malignant	bösartig (Tumor)
mallow	Malve
marigold	Ringelblume
marshmallow	Eibisch
masculine	männlich
matter	Eiter
meadow saffron	Herbstzeitlose
meal	Mahlzeit

measles	Masern
measuring spoonful	Messlöffel
medical	medizinisch Arzneimittel
medicament	Arzneimittel
medication	Verordnung, Medikamente,
medicine	Arzneimittel
melissa	Melisse
meningitis	Hirnhautentzündung
mental	geistig, seelisch
metabolism	Stoffwechsel
middle finger	Mittelfinger
migraine	Migräne
milk	Milch
mineral substances	Mineralstoffe
mistletoe	Mistel
mix	mischen
mixture	Mixtur
Monday	Montag
mononucleosis	Pfeiffersches Drüsenfieber
moustache	Schnurrbart
mouth	Mund
mouthwash	Mundwasser
mucus	Schleim
mucous membrane	Schleimhaut
mull bandage	Mullbinde
mumps	Mumps
muscle	Muskel
mute	stumm
myrrh	Myrrhe
napkin	Windel
nappy	Windel
nasal bone	Nasenbein
nasal cavity	Nasenhöhle
nausea	Übelkeit
navel	Nabel
neck	Hals
nephritis	Nierenentzündung
nervous system	Nervensystem
neurologist	Neurologe
nipple	Brustwarze (BE), Sauger für Babyflasche (AE)
nose	Nase
nose drops	Nasentropfen
nose gel	Nasengel
nose ointment	Nasensalbe
nose spray	Nasenspray
nosebleed	Nasenbluten
nostril	Nasenloch
not having breakfasted	auf nüchternen Magen
not to be taken	nicht einnehmen
nourish	nähren, pflegen
nurse	Krankenschwester, -pfleger
nursing	Pflege
nursing home	Pflegeheim
nutmeg	Muskatnuss
oats (Pl.)	Hafer
oculist	Augenarzt
odour	Geruch
ointment	Salbe
onion	Zwiebel
operate on s. th.	etw. operieren
operation	Operation
order	bestellen
organ	Organ
organ of balance	Gleichgewichtsorgan
orthopaedist	Orthopäde
OTC-drug	verschreibungsfreies Medikament
out of children's reach, of reach of children	außerhalb der Reichweite von Kindern
out of direct sunlight	vor Licht geschützt
outpatient	ambulante(r) Patient(in)
overweight	übergewichtig
pacifier	Schnuller (AE)
paediatrician	Kinderarzt

pain	Schmerz
pain-killer	Schmerzmittel
painful	schmerzhaft
palate	Gaumen
pale	blass
pancreas	Bauchspeicheldrüse
paralysis	Lähmung
parting	Scheitel
paste	Paste
patient	Patient
pepper	Pfeffer
peppermint	Pfefferminze
period pains	Menstruationsbeschwerden
perm(anent wave)	Dauerwelle
pertussis	Keuchhusten
pharmacist	Apotheker
pharmacology	Pharmakologie
pharmacopoeia	Arzneibuch
pharmacy	Apotheke
physician	Arzt
piles	Hämorrhoiden
pill	Tablette, Pille
pimple	Pickel
plantain	Wegerich
plasma lipid concentration	Blutfettwerte
plaster	Pflaster
pneumonia	Lungenentzündung
poison	Gift
poisonous	giftig
polio(myelitis)	Kinderlähmung
pollen	Pollen
popper	Druckknopf
poppy	Mohn
potato	Kartoffel
powder	Pulver, Puder
powder mixture	Pulvermischung
powdered	in Pulverform
powdered milk	Milchpulver
practice	Praxis
precaution	Vorsichtsmaßnahme

pregnancy	Schwangerschaft
pregnant	schwanger
prepare	zubereiten, vorbereiten
prescribe	verschreiben
prescription	Rezept
press stud	Druckknopf
prophylactic	vorbeugend, Prophylaktikum
protect	schützen
psychiatric treatment	psychiatrische Behandlung
psychiatrist	Psychiater
puberty	Pubertät
pupil	Pupille
pus	Eiter
radius	Speiche
rash	Ausschlag
raspberry	Himbeere
ready for use	gebrauchsfertig
recommend	empfehlen
recover	sich erholen
rectal ointment	Rektal-Salbe
reddening	Erröten
refresh	erfrischen
refreshing	erfrischend
refrigerator	Kühlschrank
regulation	Regulierung
relief	Erleichterung
remedy	Heilmittel
research	Forschung
resistant	widerstandsfähig
retardation capsules	Retardkapseln
rheumatism	Rheumatismus
rhubarb	Rhabarber
rib	Rippe
ring finger	Ringfinger
rinse	spülen
risk factor	Risikofaktor
roller	Lockenwickler
rose	Rose

rose-hip	Hagebutte
rosemary	Rosmarin
rub (in)	(ein)reiben
run a high temperature	Fieber haben
rupture of a muscle fibre	Muskelfaserriss
rye	Roggen
safety pin	Sicherheitsnadel
saffron	Safran
sage	Salbei
Saturday	Samstag
saw	Säge
scalp	Kopfhaut
scarlet fever	Scharlach
scent	Duft
sciatica	Ischias
scientific	wissenschaftlich
scissors	Schere
sea-sickness	Seekrankheit
seaweed	Tang
secrete	absondern
sedative	Beruhigungsmittel
see the doctor	zum Arzt gehen
senna	Sennespflanze
sense of taste	Geschmackssinn
sensitive	empfindlich
shake – shook – shaken	schütteln
shave	Rasur
shin (-bone)	Schienbein
shine	Glanz
shiver	zittern
shivering fit	Schüttelfrost
short-sighted	kurzsichtig
shoulder	Schulter
shoulder-blade	Schulterblatt
sick	krank
sickness	Krankheit, Übelkeit
side effect	Nebenwirkung
sign	Zeichen
sinew	Sehne
sinuses	Stirnhöhlen
sinusitis	Stirnhöhlenkatarrh
sip	in kleinen Schlucken trinken
skeleton	Skelett, Knochengerüst
skin	Haut
skin abrasion	Hautabschürfung
skull	Schädel
sleeping pill	Schlaftablette
sleeplessness	Schlaflosigkeit
small intestine	Dünndarm
small pox	Pocken
smoke	rauchen
sneeze	niesen
soft gelatine capsules	Weich(gelatine)kapsel
sole	Sohle
solution	Lösung
sore	wund
soreness	Schmerz, Wundsein
spa	Kurort
speak – spoke – spoken	sprechen
speedy recovery	gute Besserung
spice	Gewürz
spine	Wirbelsäule
splay feet	Spreizfüße
spleen	Milz
split ends	gespaltene Spitzen
spot	Fleck
sprain	verstauchen, Verstauchung
spray	Spray
sprinkle	streuen
starch	Stärke
steep	(Tee) ziehen lassen
sterile	steril
sterilizing tablet	Sterilisiertablette
sticking plaster	Wundpflaster
stiffness	Steifheit
sting – stung – stung	stechen

stinging nettle	Brennessel
stir	rühren
stitches in the side	Seitenstechen
stomach	Magen
stomachache	Bauchschmerzen
strain	zerren
strawberry	Erdbeere
stroke	Schlag(anfall)
sublingual tablet	Sublingualtablette
suck	lutschen
suffer from	leiden an
sugar content	Zuckerspiegel
sunbathe	sonnenbaden
sunburn	Sonnenbrand
Sunday	Sonntag
sunstroke	Sonnenstich
suntan	Sonnenbräune
suppository	Zäpfchen
suppuration	Eiterung
surgeon	Chirurg
surgical spirit	Wundbenzin
suspension	Suspension
swallow	schlucken
sweat	schwitzen
swell – swelled – swollen	schwellen
symptom	Symptom
syrup	Sirup
tablespoonful	Esslöffel...
tablet	Tablette
tablet for insomnia	Schlaftablette
take	(ein)nehmen
take a seat	Platz nehmen
take care of	achtgeben auf
take to excess	im Übermaß nehmen
taste	schmecken
taste buds	Geschmacksknospen
tea	Tee
tea bag	Teeaufgußbeutel
tear – tore – torn	reißen
teaspoonful	Teelöffel...
teat (BE)	Sauger (für Babyflasche)
temperature	Temperatur
temple	Schläfe
tendon	Sehne
tetanus	Wundstarrkrampf
thermometer	Thermometer
thick	dick
thigh	Oberschenkel
thin	dünn
third finger	Ringfinger
throat	Hals, Rachen
thrombosis (thromboses)	Thrombose(n)
thumb	Daumen
Thursday	Donnerstag
thyme	Thymian
thyroid	Schilddrüse
tibia	Schienbein
tight	gespannt
tightly closed	dicht verschlossen
tincture	Tinktur
tired	müde
tissue	Gewebe
toe	Zehe
tongue	Zunge
tonsillitis	Mandelentzündung
tonsils	Mandeln
tooth – teeth	Zahn – Zähne
toothache	Zahnschmerzen
toothbrush	Zahnbürste
toothpaste	Zahnpasta
toxic	toxisch, giftig
tranquillizer	Beruhigungsmittel
travel-sickness	Reiseübelkeit
treat	behandeln
triangular bandage	Dreiecktuch
tropical	tropisch
trunk	Rumpf
tuberculosis	Tuberkulose
Tuesday	Dienstag
tumeric	Gelbwurz
tummy	Magen

tumour	Tumor
tweezers	Pinzette
two tablespoonfuls	zwei Esslöffel
two tablespoons full of syrup	zwei Esslöffel Saft
typhoid (fever)	Typhus
typhus	Fleckfieber
ulcer	Geschwür
ulna	Elle
unconsciousness	Bewusstlosigkeit
undiluted	unverdünnt
upper arm	Oberarm
uvula	Gaumenzäpfchen
vaccination	Impfung
vaginal cream	Vaginalcreme
vaginal suppositories	Vaginalzäpfchen
valerian	Baldrian
varicose veins	Krampfadern
vein	Vene
venereal disease	Geschlechtskrankheit
vermouth	Wermut-Wein
vertebra	Wirbel
vertebral column	Wirbelsäule
vial	Injektionsflasche
viral	Virus-
virus	Virus
vitamin	Vitamin
vomit	erbrechen
waist	Taille
walnut	Walnuss
wart	Warze
washing	Spüllösung
waterproof	wasserfest
weak	schwach
weariness	Müdigkeit, Mattigkeit
Wednesday	Mittwoch
wet	nass
wheat	Weizen
wheelchair	Rollstuhl
wholemeal cereals	Vollkorngetreide
whooping cough	Keuchhusten
wide	breit
willow	Weide
windpipe	Luftröhre
woodruff	Waldmeister
wormwood	Wermut
worry	sich Sorgen machen
wrap	einpacken
wrapping	Verpackung
wrinkle	Falte
wrist	Handgelenk
X-ray department	Röntgenabteilung
yarrow	Schafgarbe
yellow fever	Gelbfieber

7.4. List of irregular verbs

infinitive	simple past	past participle	German
to **be**	**was/were**	**been**	sein
to **beat**	**beat**	**beaten**	besiegen, schlagen
to **become**	**became**	**become**	werden
to **break**	**broke**	**broken**	brechen
to **bring**	**brought**	**brought**	bringen
to **build**	**built**	**built**	bauen
to **burn**	**burned/burnt**	**burned/burnt**	brennen
to **buy**	**bought**	**bought**	kaufen
to **catch**	**caught**	**caught**	fangen
to **choose**	**chose**	**chosen**	(aus)wählen
to **cling**	**clung**	**clung**	(sich) festhalten
to **come**	**came**	**come**	kommen
to **cut**	**cut**	**cut**	schneiden
to **deal** (with)	**dealt**	**dealt**	(be)handeln
to **do**	**did**	**done**	tun, machen
to **draw**	**drew**	**drawn**	zeichnen
to **dream**	**dreamed/dreamt**	**dreamed/dreamt**	träumen
to **drink**	**drank**	**drunk**	trinken
to **drive**	**drove**	**driven**	fahren
to **eat**	**ate**	**eaten**	essen
to **fall**	**fell**	**fallen**	fallen
to **feed**	**fed**	**fed**	füttern
to **feel**	**felt**	**felt**	(sich) fühlen
to **find**	**found**	**found**	finden
to **forget**	**forgot**	**forgotten**	vergessen
to **get**	**got**	**got**	(be)kommen; werden
to **give**	**gave**	**given**	geben
to **go**	**went**	**gone**	gehen
to **grow**	**grew**	**grown**	wachsen
to **have**	**had**	**had**	haben
to **hear**	**heard**	**heard**	hören
to **hit**	**hit**	**hit**	schlagen; treffen
to **hold**	**held**	**held**	halten
to **hurt**	**hurt**	**hurt**	verletzen, weh tun
to **keep**	**kept**	**kept**	behalten; weiter machen
to **know**	**knew**	**known**	wissen
to **lay**	**laid**	**laid**	(etw.) legen
to **learn**	**learned/learnt**	**learned/learnt**	lernen

infinitive	simple past	past participle	German
to **leave**	**left**	**left**	(ver)lassen
to **let**	**let**	**let**	lassen
to **lie**	**lay**	**lain**	liegen
to **lose**	**lost**	**lost**	verlieren
to **make**	**made**	**made**	machen
to **mean**	**meant**	**meant**	bedeuten; meinen
to **meet**	**met**	**met**	(sich) treffen
to **pay**	**paid**	**paid**	zahlen
to **put**	**put**	**put**	stellen, legen, setzen
to **read**	**read**	**read**	lesen
to **run**	**ran**	**run**	rennen, laufen
to **say**	**said**	**said**	sagen
to **see**	**saw**	**seen**	sehen
to **sell**	**sold**	**sold**	verkaufen
to **send**	**sent**	**sent**	schicken
to **set**	**set**	**set**	setzen, legen, stellen
to **shake**	**shook**	**shaken**	schütteln
to **shine**	**shone**	**shone**	scheinen, glänzen
to **show**	**showed**	**shown**	zeigen
to **shut**	**shut**	**shut**	schließen
to **sit**	**sat**	**sat**	sitzen
to **sleep**	**slept**	**slept**	schlafen
to **smell**	**smelled/smelt**	**smelled/smelt**	riechen
to **speak**	**spoke**	**spoken**	sprechen
to **spell**	**spelled/spelt**	**spelled/spelt**	buchstabieren
to **spend**	**spent**	**spent**	ausgeben; verbringen
to **stand**	**stood**	**stood**	stehen
to **swim**	**swam**	**swum**	schwimmen
to **take**	**took**	**taken**	nehmen
to **teach**	**taught**	**taught**	lehren
to **tell**	**told**	**told**	sagen, erzählen
to **think**	**thought**	**thought**	denken
to **throw**	**threw**	**thrown**	werfen
to **understand**	**understood**	**understood**	verstehen
to **wake**	**woke**	**woken**	aufwachen; wecken
to **wear**	**wore**	**worn**	tragen, anhaben
to **win**	**won**	**won**	gewinnen
to **write**	**wrote**	**written**	schreiben

Appendix | Anhang

8

8. Appendix

8.1. Medical care in Great Britain

The National Health Service was established in 1948. Today most doctors are employed by the NHS and most hospitals are run by trusts, which are funded by the state but control their own budget.
The NHS provides free medical treatment for all people who live in Great Britain or happen to be staying there. Someone who wants to take advantage of the NHS has to register with a GP (general practitioner) who is in practice in his or her area. He will send a patient to a specialist or to hospital, if necessary. Most patients have to pay a small contribution for prescriptions, false teeth and spectacles. Concessions are made for people on social security, expectant mothers, children and people over 60 or with special needs. It is, however, not possible for the patient to choose a particular surgeon for an operation. The cost of the National Health Service is met mainly from taxation, but also from national insurance contributions.

Although the NHS provides excellent medical attention, some people prefer to be private patients. They expect prompt treatment and may have more choice of consultant. Private consultations have to be paid for by the patients. Thus there are some doctors who run private practices and others who work part-time for the NHS and charge fees to treat private patients, as well. Some hospitals have a small number of additional beds for fee-paying patients. There are a number of hospitals, which are independent of the NHS.

8.2. Medical care in the USA

For the most part, medical care in the USA is of high quality. A number of university hospitals, clinics, and health care professionals are sought out by patients from all over the world, and many specialists enjoy good reputations. There is a sufficient number of hospitals, many of which are run privately.

Getting proper medical attention can be complicated, however, due to the broad range of insurance options and the large population of uninsured. In large cities, where the standard of living is often higher, health care tends to be more expensive, and overcrowdedness and long waits in emergency situations can pose problems. The organisation of medical care in the United States is completely different from that in Great Britain or Germany. There are many types of health plans, but no standard system, no National Health Service nor compulsory health insurance. Doctors' fees, hospital costs, and prescription drug prices vary and can be quite high.

Many Americans are without insurance if it is not supplied by their employers. In fact, employers are not required to carry such insurance on all employees. If health insurance is provided, it generally covers 80% of the actual costs. Some workers and their families, notably those in labor unions, are covered by group health plans financed by employers or jointly by workers and employers.

Under certain circumstances, a person can be eligible for goverment-provided medicaid or medicare.

MEDICAID helps people who depend on public welfare and families whose members are disabled.

MEDICARE is availabe to senior citizens. But even they have to pay part of the costs themselves. Those with financial means often take out additional private insurance to cover extra expenses not covered by Medicaid or Medicare.